For the Health of a Nation

A Shared Responsibility

Report of the National Leadership
Commission on Health Care

For the Health of a Nation

A Shared Responsibility

**Report of the National Leadership
Commission on Health Care**

Health Administration Press Perspectives
Ann Arbor, Michigan
1989

94   93   92   91   90   5   4   3   2

Library of Congress Cataloging-in-Publication Data
National Leadership Commission on Health Care (U.S.).
    For the health of a nation : a shared responsibility / report of the National Leadership Commission on Health Care.
    p. cm.
    "January 1989."
    Bibliography: p.
    ISBN 0-910701-51-2
    1. Medical care—United States.   2. Medical care—United States—Finance.   I. Title.
    [DNLM: 1. Delivery of Health Care—United States.   2. Health Services Accessibility—United States.   3. Quality of Health Care—United States.   W 84 AA1 N17f]
RA445.N34   1989   362. 1'0973—dc20 DNLM/DLC for Library of Congress 89-11013 CIP

Health Administration Press
A division of the Foundation of the
    American College of Healthcare Executives
1021 East Huron Street
Ann Arbor, Michigan 48104-9990
(313) 764-1380

The National Leadership Commission
    on Health Care
555 13th Street, N.W.
Washington, D.C. 20004
(202) 637-6832

Table of Contents

Appendixes:

The National Leadership Commission on Health Care: Member List

HONORARY CO-CHAIRS

Former President Jimmy Carter
Former President Gerald Ford
Former President Richard M. Nixon

CO-CHAIRS

The Honorable Robert D. Ray, LL.B., President and Chief Executive
Officer, Blue Cross and Blue Shield of Iowa
The Honorable Paul G. Rogers, J.D., Attorney, Hogan & Hartson

PRESIDENT

Henry E. Simmons, M.D., M.P.H., F.A.C.P., Visiting Research Professor,
George Washington University

COMMISSION MEMBERS

Morris B. Abram, J.D., Attorney, Paul, Weiss, Rifkind, Wharton &
Garrison
Stuart Altman, Ph.D., Dean, Florence Heller School, Brandeis
University
William F. Buehler, Group Vice President—Human Resources, AT&T

ADVISORY GROUP

David Banta, M.D., Health Council, The Hague

Steven C. Beering, M.D., President, Purdue University

Charles R. Buck, Jr., Sc.D., Staff Executive, Health Care Programs, General Electric Company

Roger Bulger, M.D., President, Association of Academic Health Centers

Guido Calabresi, LL.B., Dean, Yale University Law School

Thomas Chalmers, M.D., Distinguished Physician, Veterans Administration

The Honorable Clark Clifford, J.D., Attorney, Clifford & Warnke

William Foege, M.D., Executive Director, Task Force for Child Survival

Rev. Theodore M. Hesburgh, C.S.C., President Emeritus, University of Notre Dame

The Honorable Carla Hills, LL.B., United States Trade Representative

John Hogness, M.D., Former President, Association of Academic Health Centers

The Honorable Barbara Jordan, J.D., Professor, L.B.J. School of Public Affairs, University of Texas

Catherine E. McDermott, President, Grant Makers in Health

Michael Maccoby, Ph.D., Director, Program on Technology, Public Policy & Human Development, John F. Kennedy School of Government, Harvard University

Dennis O'Leary, M.D., President, Joint Commission on Accreditation of Healthcare Organizations

Paul H. O'Neill, Chairman & Chief Executive Officer, Aluminum Company of America

Robert G. Petersdorf, M.D., President, Association of American Medical Colleges

Arnold S. Relman, M.D., Editor-in-Chief, *The New England Journal of Medicine*

The Honorable Elliot Richardson, LL.B., Attorney, Milbank, Tweed, Hadley & McCloy

Lewis Thomas, M.D., President Emeritus, Memorial Sloan-Kettering Cancer Center

EXECUTIVE DIRECTOR

Margaret M. Rhoades, Ph.D.

RESEARCH STAFF

Anne K. (Burns) Gauthier, Senior Researcher
Robin J. Strongin, Research Analyst
Jude Payne, Research Analyst
Jeff Stryker, Research Analyst
Joy Garney, Executive Assistant
Amanda M. Hock, Research Assistant
Beverly Nissenbaum, Research Assistant
Phyllis A. Anderson, Secretary

Foreword

THE PURPOSE

The National Leadership Commission on Health Care was formed in 1986 by a group of concerned citizens to propose workable solutions to the three major problems in health care: cost, quality, and access to care. This private sector group determined at the outset to establish a non-prejudicial forum to examine these issues and develop policy recommendations to meet the nation's health care needs into the next century. The Commission was composed of leaders from the major participants in the health care system and sought to develop consensus positions about the problems facing this system and the possible solutions to these problems.

In a system as complex as health care, it would be very difficult for any one study to examine all its elements critically. The Commission decided to concentrate on the three most central critical issues of cost, quality, and access. Fortunately, other groups in and out of government are examining important aspects of our health care system which we have not touched on. These efforts include the Physician Payment Review Commission, the Department of Health and Human Services (HHS) study of the nursing shortage, the HHS Preventive Medicine Task Force, and several studies on medical education sponsored by private foundations, either just completed or about to begin. When results of these studies become available, they could be integrated into our recommendations so that an even more comprehensive national approach can be considered. In the meantime, we feel our report and recommendations can be considered separately, and we hope action will begin on the fundamental reforms we recommend.

The Commission aimed to shape a workable vision of a fair, affordable, high quality health care system, define the actions needed to attain that vision, and engage the participants in the health care system in the effort to bring about needed changes. In the course of its work, the Commission has benefitted from a broad spectrum of opinion and expert testimony from all segments of the health care system. Commissioners also worked continuously to inform public debate about health care issues, describing the Commission and its work to those leaders in government, the private sector, and the media interested in improving our health care system.

THE PROCESS

The Commission brought together a distinguished group of leaders from many areas—health care, business, law, economics, politics, ethics, and labor. The Commissioners are drawn from groups that traditionally supported conflicting positions, and it was necessary first to develop a common understanding of the issues and a shared language.

To move beyond narrow institutional interests, Commissioners were encouraged to envision the kind of health care system that would serve us well in the twenty-first century. Convinced that government could not solve the complex problems by itself, and that all the key private participants had to join in the effort, the Commissioners responded to the challenge.

The only atmosphere in which effective consideration of the issues could take place was a "no-fault" environment. An analysis of the problems in health care led quickly to an understanding by the Commissioners that blame could not, and indeed should not, be laid at anyone's door.

In his role as facilitator of the Commission's meetings, Michael Maccoby of the Kennedy School of Government at Harvard University began the first full Commission meeting in the fall of 1986 by asking each Commissioner to state as a citizen, not as a representative of an organization, what he or she considered the most important health care issues before the United States. Three issues emerged clearly from the discussion: access to health care for all Americans, cost control, and the quality of care.

In the frank discussion that followed, strong opinions were transformed into questions that could be researched. Unlike some commissions for which the staff does the thinking and commissioners decide if it sounds good, the National Leadership Commission was a working, thinking, debating group of dedicated people. The staff provided participants with a constant flow of information and, at the direction of the Commission, periodically analyzed and summarized the issues. At least twenty Commissioners and Advisers attended each of the meetings that stretched from the fall of 1986 through December of 1988.

The first phase of the work consisted of a series of meetings to explore the nature and size of the problems in health care access, cost, and quality. Commissioners volunteered to serve on working groups on each topic. They conducted research on the problems in each area, with the help of expert witnesses, and brought their findings back to the committee of the whole. A series of meetings of the full Commission then considered these problems and developed a position which was released to the public as the Commission's interim statement of June 1987.

During its second phase, the Commission held six one- to two-day workshops to consider strategies for solving the problems we had identified. These workshops were held against the backdrop of a basic understanding that the problems of access, cost, and quality were inextricably intertwined. To address any one issue effectively, all three had to be tackled. Each workshop posed a strategic "how" question, such as, "How can we improve the appropriateness and effectiveness of our health care?" Outside experts made presentations to Commissioners at the workshops, which were open to the public and attracted many additional participants. In between Commission workshops, some Commissioners and Advisers met frequently in small, informal groups. During the past two years, over twenty such sessions have been held.

After developing a vision of the kind of system it wanted to create, the Commission developed policy proposals which could be continuously evaluated in terms of whether they really moved the system toward that vision.

The Commission believes that the vitality and quality of the health care system require not only financial resources but also a developing clinical science, a growing competence in the management of services, and freedom from over-control and chilling litigation. The Commissioners propose a system that can continually improve itself and be efficient enough not to overburden those who deliver and pay for care.

While all Commissioners agreed on the nature of the problem and supported the vision presented in this report, votes on final recommendations revealed some disagreements about the policy steps which would best resolve the problems and enable us to move toward that vision. During Commission retreats, it became clear that there were many different views represented around the table. Reflecting these differences, this report includes discussion of the reasoning behind different alternatives to controlling costs, as well as comments and dissenting views from several Commissioners (see Appendix G).

THE PEOPLE

The Commission is honored that the three former Presidents of the United States, Jimmy Carter, Gerald Ford, and Richard M. Nixon, agreed to serve as honorary co-chairs of the Commission. The Co-chairmen of the Commission provided strong leadership, a dose of political reality, and their critical consensus-building skills to the effort. Co-chairs Paul G. Rogers, former member of Congress (Democrat from Florida) from 1961 to 1979, and Robert D. Ray, former Governor (Republican from Iowa) from 1969 to 1983, represented in the leadership of the Commission its bipartisan nature. Henry E. Simmons, M.D., M.P.H., F.A.C.P., served as President.

The Commission includes leaders of American health care, business, labor, and public policy. They have all spent many years participating in the planning, providing, and paying for health care in this country. They have given the Commission enormous amounts of time, boundless energy, and, in many cases, the technical and financial support of their organizations. Several Commissioners stepped forward to lead meetings and workshops. Stuart Altman, Dean of the Florence Heller School at Brandeis University, led two of the day-long meetings of the Commission on alternative strategies with tremendous skill, knowledge, and unfailing good humor. Harry Garber, Vice Chairman of Equitable, and John Sweeney, President of the Service Employees International Union, chaired the workgroup on the uninsured and underinsured. Robert Gaynor, retired Group Vice President–Planning of AT&T, chaired the workgroup on responsibilities and access. Dr. Edmund Pellegrino, Director of the Kennedy Institute of Ethics at Georgetown University, and C.B. Rogers, Jr., President and Chief Operating Officer of Equifax, Inc., chaired the workgroup on cost and quality.

The Advisory Group includes men and women who have been leaders in the health and public policy fields for decades. Their wise counsel has helped to guide the course of our work, and we are grateful. The work of the Commission has been ably assisted by more people than we can readily name. A group of Technical Advisers, comprised of leaders of the medical specialty societies, the American Nurses' Association, and the Mayo Clinic, have frequently given the Commission the benefit of their perspective on issues the Commission has addressed. We are particularly indebted to Dr. Richard Southby, Chairman of the Department of Health Services Administration at George Washington University, for providing space and support for the start-up phase of the Commission. We are indebted to the law firm of Hogan and Hartson for the many services they provided the Commission; Commission staff moved into space at the firm in September of 1986.

Immeasurable support has been provided to the Commission by leading experts in the health policy field. Several of them wrote excellent background papers for the Commission. David Mechanic of the Institute for Health, Health Care Policy, and Aging Research at Rutgers University wrote "The Doctor-Patient Relationship: Traditions, Transitions and Tension" in 1986. Rashi Fein, Professor at the Harvard University Medical School, wrote "Medical Costs" in January 1987. Dr. David Eddy and John Billings, both of the Center for Health Policy Research and Education at Duke University, wrote "The Quality of Medical Evidence and Medical Practice" in May 1987. Dr. John Wennberg of the Dartmouth University Medical School wrote "The Medical Care Outcome Problem: An Agenda for Action" in May 1987. Lawrence S. Lewin, President of the Lewin/ICF Group, wrote "Cost Containment until Today: Lessons for Tomorrow" in May 1988. A listing of the many important figures in government and the private sector who spoke before the Commission is found in Appendix B.

The Lewin/ICF Group contributed critical background analyses of the financing, cost elements, and organization of the Commission's models for the future. Their path-breaking work, led by Lawrence S. Lewin and John Shiels, was noteworthy for the clarity of its writing, the cogency of its argument, and the timeliness of its delivery. Paul Campbell of the Lash Group contributed important and clearly written analyses of the Commission's models. Hill and Knowlton, Seltzer Daley Companies, and the Washington law firm of Arent, Fox, Kintner, Plotkin & Kahn provided assistance at the outset.

The Commission was ably assisted by a small staff. Margaret M. Rhoades served from September 1986 as Executive Director. Anne K. Burns was Senior Researcher. For the first year, Jeff Stryker served as Research Analyst. Jude Payne and Robin J. Strongin were Research Analysts for two years. Joy Garney acted as Executive Assistant and Amanda Hock as Research Assistant, following Beverly Nissenbaum as Research Assistant and Phyllis Anderson as secretary. David Riley edited the manuscript. The entire staff performed with skill, presenting the Commission with carefully chosen and articulated material, planning the workshops and meetings, and supporting the research and writing effort with unfailing good humor.

The Commission

Executive Summary

Formed in 1986 by a group of concerned citizens to address the three major problems of cost, quality, and access to health care, the National Leadership Commission on Health Care proposes a major restructuring of the nation's health care system. The Commission's proposal provides universal access to a basic level of health services; it controls escalating costs through use of economic leverage in the purchase of care, economic incentives including cost sharing, and through practice guidelines to encourage appropriate care and eliminate unnecessary care, based on greatly expanded research on the quality and appropriateness of health care. The Commission believes that reducing unnecessary procedures will both contain costs and improve the quality of health care. Its malpractice reform recommendations will also help contain costs and improve quality.

The Commission brought together a distinguished group of leaders from many areas—health care, business, law, economics, politics, ethics, and labor. The Commission sought to develop a clear sense of the scope of the problems in health care, a vision to reach for, and workable solutions to bring us closer to that vision. It released an interim statement in June, 1987, outlining its view of the seriousness of the problems.

During its deliberations, the Commission agreed on a vision of a better health care system in the 21st century, one which promotes preventive care and healthy lifestyles, and establishes an innovative, efficient health care system that provides universal access to a basic level of appropriate, affordable care. The system would encourage personal responsibility for choosing good health and appropriate treatment, support a strong doctor-patient relationship, and promote a public-private partnership to control costs and improve the quality of care. It also proposes specific solutions to the malpractice crisis.

PROBLEMS WITH THE CURRENT HEALTH CARE SYSTEM

The American health care system has done a remarkable job in many ways in providing health care to the American people. American medicine has long been a leader in the field, making significant contributions in the form of important new technologies to prevent and treat disease. Public and private insurance programs combine to protect most Americans against devastating losses at vulnerable times of ill health and disability. Yet millions of Americans are disenfranchised, encountering barriers of entry to the health care system. Health care costs are escalating so rapidly that many payers have become alarmed at the upward spiral. And fundamental questions are now being asked about the quality, appropriateness and uncertainties of care being delivered.

Serious strains in the system are raising the frustrations of all who participate in it. Physicians are concerned about outside parties intruding on their clinical decisions and damaging the doctor-patient relationship. Hospitals find it increasingly difficult to cope with pressures for cost containment and with rapidly changing laws and regulations. Government and major private payers are trying with limited success to control rising costs. Patients are faced with higher costs, but they don't see care improving sufficiently to justify their increasing payments—and they continue to present the system with ever-increasing demands. Such strains in the health care system will be exacerbated by the rapid aging of the population, the AIDS epidemic, and the continuing technology explosion, which spawns more and more new treatments, that, though often beneficial, are also costly.

These problems grew out of the postwar period, which ushered in wonder drugs, sophisticated medical technology and the expansion of health insurance to cover the majority of the population. With the adoption of the Medicare and Medicaid programs in 1965, 85 percent of the population had some form of health insurance, leaving the consumers of health care shielded from, and thus much less sensitive to, cost increases than consumers in other sectors of the economy.

Cost

These developments have led to increases in health care expenditures that far outstrip general inflation rates. Factors fueling the cost increases include general inflation, accelerated inflation in medical care prices, the aging of the population, patient demand, increasing physician supply, the use of inappropriate care, the practice of defensive medicine, and advances in medical science leading to expensive new technologies—all compounded by the inherently inflationary ways in which most care is financed and delivered. The health care sector is one of the three largest sectors of the economy, so that inability to control costs in this area will have an important negative impact on the economy as a whole. Thus, serious concerns exist among government, American industry, and the American people about the cost issue. Furthermore, continued cost escalation in light of constrained resources could ultimately compromise everyone's access to care and further adversely affect its quality. To prevent this, it is imperative to bring costs under control.

Americans spent $550 billion on health care in 1988, over 11 percent of GNP, far more than any other country. If these trends continue, costs will double by 1995 and triple by the turn of the century, hitting $1.5 trillion in the year 2000. In that year, health care will consume 15 percent of GNP, and this country will spend $5,551 on health care for every American man, woman, and child. The National Economic Commission estimates that if present trends continue, by the year 2005 the Medicare program alone will exceed in size either the Social Security or the defense budgets.

As a result, cost containment has become a rallying cry in both the private and public sectors. The federal government has enacted the prospective payment system (PPS) for hospitals, setting payment in advance according to a patient's diagnosis. Some state governments have instituted closely regulated global budgeting for hospitals and tight control on new construction. Private payers have turned to managed care mechanisms, such as health maintenance organizations (HMOs), as a way to hold down costs, Such efforts have successfully reduced inpatient hospital use, but they have also shifted costs to the outpatient setting, where costs have continued to rise rapidly.

Access

Increasing costs are accompanied by another disturbing development: growing numbers of people without health insurance, or with inadequate health insurance, and therefore without good access to health care. Financial strains on the Medicaid program mean that it now covers only 45 percent of those in need. Today about 37 million Americans lack insurance. A third of the uninsured are children. Perhaps an equal number have very inadequate coverage. Thus one out of every four Americans may be either uninsured or seriously underinsured. These people tend not to seek help until they are quite sick, which makes them more of a burden on the health care system than they would otherwise be.

Quality

Quality of care is the third area of major concern. We have insufficient information on the quality and outcomes of medical services and insufficient means of monitoring the quality of care and fostering its improvement. Recent studies have heightened this concern, citing large regional variations in the use of some medical services that do not seem to be based on differences in medical need. Over the past two years, there has been a steady drumbeat of stories detailing the percentage of unnecessary and equivocal care in the use of one procedure after another. It has become clear to many experts that this is no longer a problem isolated to a few specialities but rather is generic to the health care of the nation. The sad fact is that our quality control systems are at best rudimentary. Hospitals, for example, have traditionally focused only on how care is delivered; they have just begun to measure the impact of that care on patient outcomes. Patients also have few tools to help them assess the quality and appropriateness of their treatment.

These critical problems in cost, quality, and access to health care in America present a clear and compelling case for change. They are interrelated problems that cry out for interrelated solutions. Piecemeal approaches have not worked in the past and will not in the future. Each problem can be solved effectively only in relation to the other two. Until we can better define quality and appropriate care, we cannot really know what is worth providing access to and what is worth paying for.

The Commission's Proposal

In response to these serious problems, the Commission proposes a new public/private partnership to optimize health outcomes and the use of economic resources. This strategy is designed to control costs, define and assure universal access to a basic level of health services and improve the quality and appropriateness of care.

Under our proposal, all Americans would be required to have health insurance for a package of basic services. There are several ways in which such coverage could be secured, including employment-based coverage, personal payments, or participation in our Universal Access (UNAC) program.

Our model calls for a shared responsibility to finance care for the currently uninsured. It retains a significant role for the states and private insurance companies. It is structured to strengthen market forces and foster competition and innovation in the quality and efficient management of health care services. The plan calls for a strong education campaign to encourage patients to adopt healthy lifestyles and to inform patients and providers about guidelines for appropriate care to help them make better decisions about treatment.

The Commission's strategy has the following additional elements:

- *Expand the existing insurance system* by encouraging all employers to provide health insurance for their employees.

- *Establish a nationally determined level of basic services* of health care available to all, allowing for state variations above that level.

- *Greatly increase research on the appropriateness, effectiveness, and quality of care* and publicize the results widely to help patients, providers, and payers assess treatment.

- *Control costs by reducing the amount of inappropriate care* as a result of the expanded research and national guidelines.

- *Encourage the marketplace to work more efficiently* by using new, solid information about appropriateness, quality, and cost, and by developing more cost-effective delivery systems.

- *Develop a strong public-private partnership to improve quality and control costs* by coordinating the expanded research on appropriateness and quality and disseminating the results through health professional and other appropriate organizations.

- *Develop and continually update national guidelines* to enable practitioners, patients, and payers to make more informed decisions.

- *Expand the existing state agencies* to operate the UNAC program and negotiate fair payment to providers who serve that population.

- *Promote nationwide the current, promising state reforms in malpractice* and consider new federal initiatives if necessary.

A realistic strategy must not only deal with all three areas of cost, access, and quality; it must also engage all the parties which provide, pay for and use health care. This means that any effective system-wide solution must be a public-private partnership. The responsibility does not lie with the government alone, which pays for 40 percent of the country's health care bill, but also with private individuals and other private payers, who account for the other 60 percent.

While our systemic approach to reform is important, individual parts of the solution can be modified without endangering the integrity of the overall solution. For example, the source of the funding for improving access and expanded research could come from general revenues rather than a specific premium and fees. For illustrative purposes, our proposal sketches out the dimensions of one particular approach to funding. We recognize there are other possible approaches which could accomplish the same objectives.

Fundamental Principles

The Commission's proposal is based on seven fundamental principles which the Commission developed during its deliberations.

I. *Principle of Universal Access:*

There should be no financial barrier separating Americans in need of health care from access to available care.

II. *Principle of Fair Compensation*:

Every provider of health services in America should be adequately compensated for services rendered to patients.

III. *Principle of Clinical and Economic Freedom:*

To the maximum extent possible, without unduly compromising other important principles, health policy ought to restore clinical freedom in rendering health services and economic freedom in financing these services, within the context of adequate counter-vailing market power from those who ultimately pay for health care in America.

IV. *Principle of Shared Responsibility*:

Financial responsibility for health care for those too poor to afford it should be shared by government, individuals and employers.

V. *Principle of Individual Responsibility*:

To help achieve the goal of universal access to health care, the individual has a duty to have adequate health insurance coverage for him- or herself and dependent children.

VI. *Principle of Basic Benefits Guarantee:*

The design of a basic package of health-service benefits to which all Americans should have reliable access is ultimately a federal responsibility.

VII. *Principle of a Strong Doctor-Patient Relationship:*

Any health care system should foster the goal of protecting the integrity of the doctor-patient relationship.

The Commission's proposal builds upon the American tradition of providing private health insurance through the workplace. It is designed to encourage continued extensive reliance on that approach, without mandating that employers provide such coverage. The system thus preserves the pluralistic approach to health-care financing apparently preferred by Americans.

The National Leadership Commission does not consider it appropriate for it to establish the national basic benefits package for all Americans. The initial package would be set by enabling legislation. But the Commission strongly recommends that mental health benefits and preventive services, especially prenatal care, be included in this package.

Access to Care for All Americans

The Commission's proposal, known as the Universal Access or UNAC program, would extend health coverage to the 37 million Americans who now lack health insurance. All Americans would be covered at least for the national basic package of services. There are several ways they could obtain this coverage. Most Americans would probably continue to obtain privately-financed coverage as an employment benefit. Any American could also choose to purchase basic coverage or could supplement employer-provided coverage with personal funds. Older Americans would continue to receive Medicare coverage. Everyone else would receive coverage through the UNAC fund. The Commission proposes that all employers, and all individuals with incomes above 150 percent of the poverty level, pay a premium or a fee to finance health insurance for the uninsured. The Commission's plan uses strong incentives to encourage employers to offer coverage and to improve coverage under some existing plans. It also has provisions for all individuals who can afford to do so to pay for part of their care.

The Commission has presented a plan in its report which details how this proposal could work in practice. The Commission believes the most reasonable estimate is that about 67.9 million people will become covered under the UNAC program. If all employers chose to provide insurance rather than pay the X_1 fee, the number in the program could

Table 1: A Snap-Shot of Estimated Fees and Premiums[a] (in 1988 figures; estimates include administrative costs)

		Basic-option[b]	Low-option[b]
Pay only in absence of health insurance	X_1 fee (employer)	9.68%	8.75%
	X_2 fee (employee)	2.04%	1.85%
Everyone pays (includes health services research)	Y premium (employer)	0.68%	0.58%
	Y premium (employee)	0.66%	0.56%

[a]The X_1 fee is a percentage of wages and salaries up to $45,000. The X_2 fee and the Y premium are a percentage of adjusted gross income up to $45,000.

[b]These different benefit plans are described in Technical Appendix I and Appendix B.

be as small as 42.9 million. Estimates of the costs of various provisions of the proposal and how they would be financed are given in the full report.

The Commission's UNAC safety net system would be administered at the state level by a cooperative effort involving all stakeholders in the health care system. The federal government would provide guidelines

Figure 1: Funding Mechanism for UNAC Program

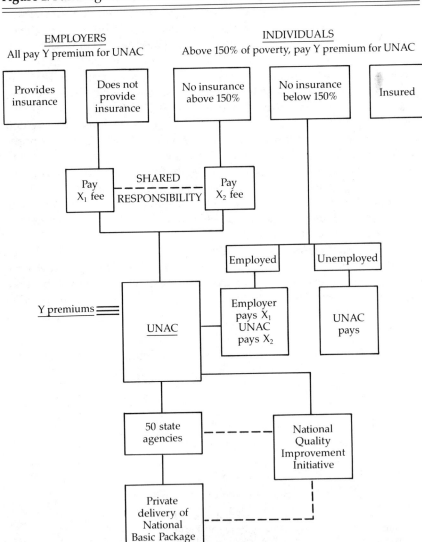

for the program designed to treat all Americans equally, regardless of location, but the program would not be centrally directed as is, for example, the Medicare program. There would be ample room for regional variations within broad federal guidelines.

In addition to a national package of basic health care benefits to which every American has access, the Commission's proposal allows the states to determine any additional benefits for their residents. The UNAC program would be administered by state agencies which would have the power to negotiate with providers and practitioners to establish the package and payment policies for UNAC beneficiaries. The Commission recommends the utilization of existing state agencies, where possible, rather than creation of a new level of bureaucracy. The Commission recommends that states broaden their agencies to include representatives of the major private stakeholders in health care—payers, practitioners, and consumers—perhaps appointed by state governors.

The Commission recognizes that it will not be easy to generate the cooperation needed to realize its goals, primarily because attitudes will have to change. But the Commission is unanimously convinced that cooperation is both desirable and possible. It is clear to the Commission from its discussions with dozens of physicians and the testimony of leaders of the professions that they are eager to play a role in this process. The Commission regards their role as essential to the success of any proposed change in health care policy.

Cost Control and Quality Improvement

The Commission's approach to cost control goes beyond the provisions summarized above. It is also inextricably linked to its proposal for improving the quality and appropriateness of health care. The Commission plan seeks to remove cross-subsidies and make explicit the cost of care for all. Some or all of the cost of providing universal access would be made up in savings resulting from more appropriate care and improved quality control. The Commission's strategy is designed to improve both the value of care and the efficiency of the systems that provide care. A marketplace approach by definition, the Commission's proposal would greatly increase information available to providers and patients on the quality and appropriateness of health care. Such information, if widely disseminated, would allow the competitive advances of the past few years to play out.

The Commission has concluded that an important level of inappropriate over- and underuse of care has been documented for some time now. The reasons for inappropriate care include the following: an incomplete and continually evolving science base for that care, often creating uncertainty about appropriateness and effectiveness in clinical decisionmaking; perverse financial incentives; seeking to meet unrealistically high patient expectations; and the malpractice crisis. In addition, systems to assure that care is provided in the best fashion are too often inadequate.

Health professionals and patients need several types of knowledge. They need to know which tests and procedures are appropriate for an individual situation. When guidelines exist for particular conditions or treatments, they need to examine the scientific basis of those guidelines to determine its adequacy. They also need more information about which medical practices are truly effective and which are not. And they need better ways to measure what happens when care is provided and how it can be more effective. This can only occur within a general understanding that each patient presents a unique set of problems.

Improving information on quality and appropriateness will have far-reaching effects. In addition to reducing the level of uncertainty, which in turn reduces unnecessary and inappropriate care, improvements in quality and appropriateness information should also help stem the tide of increasing health care costs, increase efficiency, improve the doctor-patient relationship, and reduce defensive medicine and malpractice suits. Fortunately, there is solid evidence that health care providers will use relevant, well-presented information to improve the quality and appropriateness of their care. The Commission has found that governmental agencies and private organizations with clinical expertise are actively pursuing:

1. Objective analysis of the proper use of existing and emerging approaches to diagnosis and treatment, often known as appropriateness research and technology assessment;
2. Clinical trials on the effectiveness of medical practices;
3. Research designed to understand and, where appropriate, reduce practice variation, often known as outcomes research and practice pattern monitoring;
4. Synthesis of current research and clinical experience into practical clinical practice guidelines; and
5. Development and use of clinical and organizational measures to stimulate improvement in the quality and appropriateness of care.

National Quality Improvement Initiative. The Commission has found, however, that this work is woefully underfunded. The Commission has also found lacking a process where participants can develop a nationally coordinated strategy. The Commission proposes a National Quality Improvement Initiative that would fund such work and would involve periodic collective priority setting, coordination, and progress evaluation, while maintaining decentralized activities.

The Commission's plan would raise additional funds for this important research with a supplemental fee applied to the Y premium (see chart) for both employers and individuals. We estimate that with a rate applied to both the employer and the employee Y revenue bases of about one-tenth of one percent (0.11 percent), the research fund would reach $500 million per year.

At the Commission's request, Lewin/ICF prepared a very rough estimate of potential savings that could be generated by reducing inappropriate care. Based on HCFA estimates that as much as two percentage points of the annual hospital intensity index would be influenced by practice pattern changes, the Commission's estimate suggests a potential savings of two percentage points of the currently projected growth rate of health expenditure. This means that over a four-year period, about $5.9 billion annually for Medicare Parts A and B combined could be influenced by changes in practice pattern. For national health expenditures, the figure is $84 billion for fiscal year 1990-1993, or an average of $22 billion annually that could be influenced by practice pattern changes. Using a second method of approximating the potential effects of changing practice patterns on health care costs, the Commission developed a very conservative "bottom up" estimate of potential savings from reducing inappropriate services; assuming a 4 percent growth rate in health expenditures annually, this estimate could approach $1.5 billion a year by FY 1993.

Malpractice Reform

The Commission believes that the current system of malpractice litigation against providers of health care—hospitals, physicians and nurses—impedes the delivery of economical, high-quality care to American citizens. The Commission recognizes that patients should be fully compensated for injuries resulting from negligent care, and it supports strengthening procedures to identify and correct below-standard practices, but the present system of medical malpractice litigation does not achieve either goal and has other adverse consequences as well.

Malpractice litigation has driven up the cost of medical care overall and, in some specialties, at a dramatic rate. Providers who can obtain malpractice insurance are forced to pass on its rising cost to patients (or third-party payers) through increased fees. The fear of malpractice suits encourages defensive medicine, in which providers perform additional procedures, especially diagnostic ones, principally to protect themselves against law suits. Such procedures increase both the cost of care and sometimes health risks to patients. The current system of malpractice litigation also corrodes the patient-physician relationship.

We are, therefore, convinced that the malpractice system must be reformed, and we are encouraged by the breadth of interest in reform both within the medical profession and outside it. Some promising proposals have been adopted experimentally on a state or local basis, and we strongly support continued exploration of potential solutions and the adoption of the most promising reforms at the national level. Such proposals include instituting strict criteria for expert witnesses in malpractice suits, strengthening standards of negligence, limiting punitive damages and contingency fees, and encouraging mediation and arbitration as alternatives to lawsuits for resolving disputes.

CONCLUSION

The Commission calls for a solution in three parts to a system undermined by three very serious problems. The problems are unnecessary, because we know how to solve them. They are larger than they ever needed to be because for years we understood them too little, we spent time blaming one party or another, and we did not have the scientific knowledge in some areas to respond to them. In recent years, we have found the will, we have learned that no single party is to blame, and we have developed the scientific ability to improve, to begin to close the gap between art and science that has characterized medicine for many years. There will always be some art and some uncertainty, because our science continuously stretches into new areas and because every patient presents a unique set of problems. But today we have some promising methods for reducing uncertainty. It is incumbent on us to use them and to improve them continually to advance the quality and control the cost of care.

Above all, we are hopeful. Much has happened in just the two-and-a-half short years of the life of this Commission that indicates to us that all parties involved in analyzing, delivering, paying for, and benefiting from health care in this country are anxious to become involved in a solution that works. We hope that our strategies will suggest a way.

Technical Advisers

American Academy of Family Physicians	James G. Jones, M.D. President American Academy of Family Physicians
American Academy of Pediatrics	Stanley Pappelbaum, M.D. Committee on Child Health Financing American Academy of Pediatrics
American College of Obstetricians and Gynecologists	Harry S. Jonas, M.D. Former President American College of Obstetricians and Gynecologists
American College of Physicians	John R. Ball, M.D. Executive Vice President American College of Physicians
	Roger Bulger, M.D. President Association of Academic Health Centers
	John R. Hogness, M.D. Former President Association of Academic Health Centers
American College of Radiology	Joseph Marasco, Jr., M.D. Former President American College of Radiology

American College of Surgeons

Lucian L. Leape, M.D.
Committee on Continuing
    Education
American College of Surgeons

American Nurses' Association,
    Inc.

Judith Ryan, Ph.D., R.N.
Executive Director
American Nurses' Association,
    Inc.

Mayo Clinic

Fred T. Nobrega, M.D.
Director, Health Services
    Evaluation Unit
Mayo Clinic

Acknowledgements

The Commission is grateful for the financial support and good counsel it has received from the foundations, corporations, and labor unions who have given generously in support of a uniquely American concept of public service: a group of private citizens who joined together to examine a major issue confronting the nation and did so in the public interest.

AFL-CIO
Alcoa Foundation
American Federation of State, County and Municipal Employees
AT&T Foundation
Bankers Trust (Des Moines)
CIBA-GEIGY Corporation
The Coca-Cola Foundation
E.I. du Pont de Nemours & Company
Eastman Kodak Charitable Trust
Equifax, Inc.
The Equitable Financial Companies
Ford Motor Company Fund
General Electric Foundation
General Motors Foundation
Glass, Pottery, Plastics and Allied Workers International Union
W.R. Grace Foundation, Inc.
William T. Grant Foundation
Harker's, Inc.
Hoffmann–La Roche, Inc.
HON Industries Charitable Foundation
IBM
International Union of Bricklayers and Allied Craftsmen
The Robert Wood Johnson Foundation
Life Investors Insurance Company of America

Maytag Corporation
Merck Company Foundation
Metropolitan Life Foundation
Mobil Foundation, Inc.
Peat Marwick Main and Co.
Pella Rolscreen Foundation
Perot Systems Corporation
The Pew Charitable Trusts
Pfizer, Inc.
PPG Industries Foundation
The Prudential Foundation
Rockwell International
Rogers Holdings
John Ruan Foundation Trust
The Rubbermaid Foundation
Arnold & Marie Schwartz Fund for Education and Health Research
Service Employees International Union
Squibb Corporation
3M
The Upjohn Company
USX Foundation, Inc.
Varied Investments, Inc.
Westinghouse Foundation

The views expressed in this report are those of the Commission and do not necessarily reflect those of our advisers and supporters.

The Commission's Vision of Health Care for the 21st Century

- A *healthy society* in a healthy environment.
- Universal *access to a basic level of care*, providing a range of necessary services, including preventive, acute, chronic, and mental health care.
- Vigorous *public education*, emphasizing *preventive care, healthy lifestyles*, and appropriate levels of care.
- *Appropriate care* based on general agreement, resulting from solid scientific assessments, on what procedures and technologies are considered effective.
- An innovative, efficient health care system that operates in a *culture of continuous improvement*.
- Resolution of *the malpractice crisis* so that malpractice concerns are no longer a significant consideration in health care delivery.
- *Patient contributions* to the cost of their care, although only a minimal amount for the poorest, so that patients feel individual responsibility for their care.
- *Affordable* health care.
- *Controlled costs*, emphasizing payment for appropriate, efficient care.
- A high level of *personal responsibility* for health care and for understanding the options, costs, and benefits of health care decisions.
- *A strong doctor-patient relationship* based on trust and a well-informed patient.
- A strong *public-private partnership* dedicated to expanding access, controlling costs, and improving the quality of health care.

Statement of Ethical Concerns

The Commission recognizes that ethical issues inevitably underlie any recommendations of a national health care policy; these issues recurred throughout the discussions of the Commission. Ethical issues arise because health care providers—physicians, nurses, other health professionals, and institutions—operate in a special environment. They provide goods and services for which they are compensated, like other commercial transactions, yet they have a major responsibility for the health, well-being, and the very lives of those who buy their goods and services.

This responsibility raises several ethical issues. Because health care is a special kind of universal human need associated with the vulnerability and potential exploitability of the sick person, a relationship of trust between the patient and the health care provider is central to successful care. Fidelity to that trust requires that the provider's self-interest not be the primary motive and that providers avoid conflicts between their interests and those of their patients.

Since health care is a universal need essential for people to function in society, it follows that society has an obligation to provide for access to an adequate level of care for all its people. No society can be healthy if its members are not healthy.

Providing health care differs from other commercial transactions in another important respect: medical knowledge is not proprietary information that belongs exclusively to one owner. Medical knowledge is a societal good held in trust by health care providers for the benefit of all the members of society. One could not justify having access to knowledge that could save lives or ameliorate suffering without making that knowledge available to those who need it.

Since both societal and individual resources available for health care are limited, health care providers are ethically obligated to apply medical knowledge competently and efficiently. This means that medical procedures should be carried out not only in a safe way, but that they should also meet rigorous and quantifiable standards of effectiveness. Health care providers are under a moral compulsion to manage health care resources wisely, economically, and efficiently.

Patients for their part have a moral obligation to care for their own health by eliminating deleterious lifestyles and by foregoing medical treatment when it is ineffective, particularly toward the end of life when the only effect of treatment may be to prolong dying. Society in turn has a moral obligation to help people, through education and policies of encouragement, to care for their own health. But even if such incentives do not persuade people to care for their own health, a moral society should not abandon them.

Since resources for health care are finite, major moral issues arise over the allocation of resources between health and other social goods, such as education, security, and housing. Similarly, allocating resources among health care needs also raises ethical issues concerning primary versus tertiary care, caring for the young versus the elderly, and prevention versus cure.

Rationing is clearly an ethical issue. When is it justified to ration health care? Should certain conditions be met first, such as assuring the practice of effective medicine, putting in place efficient management, and eliminating useless treatments? If these conditions are met, then other ethical issues remain, such as what principle of distribution is the most just: equity, merit, social worth, ability to pay, need? A society reveals itself in the way it distributes its resources and makes its rationing decisions and the values it uses to justify its choices.

To treat all these issues fairly, the Commission recognizes that some public forum should be found in which the public can participate in the way decisions are made to protect the common interest. There are compelling questions here for the American people to consider. Where does health care stand in the priorities of the American people? How much of society's other goods and expenditures are people willing to forego in order to obtain an adequate level of health care for all? Individual patients—and therefore, cumulatively, society—are the final decision-makers about health care policy. In a democratic society, it is the people, not organizations such as the medical profession, insurance companies, hospitals, or even the government, who must confront these moral dilemmas.

The Commission believes that the final configuration of a national health care policy will depend on the answers our society gives to the ethical issues outlined here.

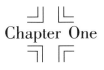

Chapter One

Problems with the Current Health Care System

The American health care[1] system has in many ways done a remarkable job in providing health care to the American people. American medicine has long been considered a leader in the field, making superb contributions in the form of important new technologies to prevent, diagnose, and treat disease. Public and private insurance programs combine to protect most Americans against devastating financial losses from ill health and disability. Yet millions of Americans are disenfranchised from our health care system, its costs are escalating at an alarming rate, and fundamental questions are being asked about the quality and appropriateness of health care.

Serious strains in the system are raising the frustrations of all who participate in it. Physicians are concerned about outside parties intruding in their clinical decisions and damaging the doctor-patient relationship. Hospitals are burdened by pressures for cost containment and rapidly changing laws and regulations. Government and major private payers are striving, with limited success, to control costs. Patients are faced with higher costs but they don't see care improving sufficiently to justify their increasing payments—and they continue to present the system with increasing demands. Such strains in the health care system will be exacerbated by the aging of the population, the AIDS epidemic, and the continuing technology explosion, which spawns more and more new treatments that, though often beneficial, are also costly.

---

[1]Throughout this report, health care is used interchangeably with medical care. We recognize that health depends on much more than medical care. Though the health care system currently focuses primarily on medical care, our goal is to strive for creation of a continuum of health services, including prevention and long-term care, coupled with a financing mechanism which encourages their optimal use.

These strains reflect the three underlying challenges which our system faces today: providing equitable access to health care, controlling its costs, and improving its quality, efficiency, and appropriateness.

HISTORICAL OVERVIEW

World War II had seen the first widespread use of a miracle drug, the antibiotic, and the years following the war witnessed a flood of new drugs and procedures from America's preeminent scientific establishment. The era of modern medicine began, following the war, with the dramatic expansion of health care professionals, hospitals, technologies, and health insurance coverage.

In a spiral of interrelated events, more physicians specialized, new technologies were developed for their use, and public expectations increased. With the adoption in 1965 of the Medicare and Medicaid programs, 85 percent of the population had some form of health insurance. In response to increasing patient demand, and stimulated by tax laws which induced employers to offer non-cash rather than cash benefits, extensive, open-ended insurance coverage burgeoned in this era.

The result of these developments was a far greater increase in health care expenditures than the major payers anticipated. In the 24 years since the passage of Medicare, national health care expenditures have increased more than ten-fold—from $41.9 billion, or 5.9 percent of GNP to $550 billion, or over 11 percent of GNP. Shielded by broad insurance coverage, patients and providers felt little need to react to rising costs.

The dramatic expansion of the early postwar era led to extensive cost containment efforts, especially over the past decade. Recently, the federal government enacted the prospective payment system (PPS) for hospitals, whereby payment amounts are set in advance according to a patient's diagnosis. Some state governments instituted global budgeting for hospitals; others placed tight controls on new construction. Private payers turned to managed care mechanisms, such as health maintenance organizations (HMOs), as a way to hold down costs. These developments reduced inpatient costs for hospitals, but shifted costs to the outpatient setting. There, increases in volume, price, and intensity of care ensured that the total costs would continue to rise rapidly.

Increasing costs have been accompanied by another troublesome development: a significant increase in the number of people without health insurance and, therefore, without good access to health care. This problem was aggravated by the deep recession in the early eighties and has not improved. Since then, the number of uninsured has increased by 50 percent. Today, about 37 million Americans lack insurance. A third of them are children. Perhaps an equal number have very inadequate coverage. That means as many as one in four Americans is either uninsured or underinsured. These people tend not to seek help until they are quite sick, which makes them an even more serious burden on the health care system than they would otherwise be.

In addition to the postwar crises of cost and access, the quality of care is a third area of major concern. It is increasingly clear that we have insufficient information on the quality, appropriateness, and outcomes of medical services and insufficient systems for monitoring the quality of care and fostering its improvement. Recent studies have heightened this concern, citing large regional variations that do not seem to be based on differences in medical need, in the use of some medical services. Over the past several years, a steady drumbeat of stories describes unnecessary or equivocal care in the use of one procedure after another. Many experts conclude that this problem is no longer isolated to a few specialties but rather is generic to the health care of the nation. (1)

These three interrelated core issues—access, cost, and quality—are described more fully below.

RAPIDLY RISING COSTS OF CARE

Overview

"Spending for medical care in the U.S. is rising so rapidly that during the 1980s it constituted the single greatest shift in spending allocation within the nation's income." (2) Costs have increased tenfold in the last 24 years and continue to rise rapidly. This increase has far outstripped the rise in inflation or rises in costs of other goods and services, continuing a pattern dating back into the 1970s. (3) If present trends continue, total costs will double in six years and triple in 12 years, hitting $1.5 trillion in the year 2000. In that year, health care will consume 15 percent of GNP, and this country will spend $5,551 on health care for every man, woman, and child. In 1987, health care costs rose 7.7 percent, although the overall inflation rate (CPI) slowed to 1.1 percent. Physician fees have increased 16 percent for each of the past six years.

We currently spend approximately 11.5 percent of our GNP on health care, much more per capita than any other nation, and our cost escalation far outstrips that of any other.

Despite 15 years of cost containment efforts by government and the private sector, health costs continue to rise rapidly. At present, there seems to be no natural limit to how high health care costs could rise.

American industry, the largest payer for health care, is experiencing major cost escalation. In light of its serious budget deficit, the Federal

Figure 1: Growth in Health Spending and GNP, Adjusted for Inflation

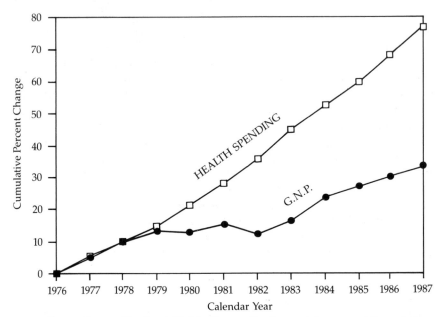

Source: Prepared by the staff of the Prospective Payment Assessment Commission, Washington, DC, Spring 1987.

government is equally concerned about massive increases in the Medicare and Medicaid budgets; National Economic Commission projections estimate that if present trends continue, by the year 2005 the Medicare program alone will exceed in size either the Social Security or Defense budgets.

The health care sector is one of the three largest sectors of the economy, so that inability to control costs in this area will have an important negative impact on the economy as a whole. Thus, serious concerns exist among government, American industry, and the American people about the cost issue. Furthermore, continued cost escalation in light of constrained resources could ultimately compromise everyone's access to care and further adversely affect its quality. To prevent this, it is imperative to bring costs under control.

Reasons for Cost Escalation

Factors fueling the cost increases include general inflation, accelerated inflation in medical care prices, the aging of the population, patient

Figure 2: International Comparisons of Health Expenditures

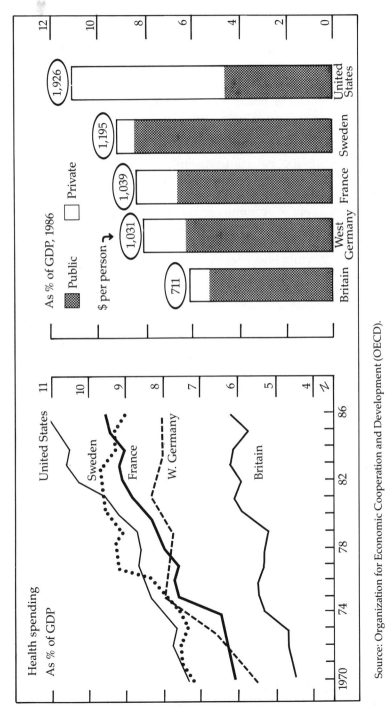

Source: Organization for Economic Cooperation and Development (OECD).

Note: For purposes of international comparison, OECD uses GDP—Gross Domestic Product—rather than GNP.

demand, increasing physician supply, the use of inappropriate care, the practice of defensive medicine, and advances in medical science leading to expensive new technologies—all compounded by the inherently inflationary ways in which most care is financed and delivered. Trends such as general economic conditions and demographic changes, while outside the control of health policy, greatly affect the country's health needs. Population growth alone will push up costs and, particularly, the needs of an aging population. More recently, AIDS has also compounded health care cost problems.

Certain unique aspects to health care make it difficult to control rising costs. Due to widespread insurance coverage, patients and providers are much less responsive to prices than are consumers and payers in other sectors of the economy. Demand is also not easily susceptible to change, since, on the one hand, physicians can create their own demand and are trained to do as much as possible for their patients, and on the other hand, patients often develop unrealistically high expectations. To the physician, the ambiguity and complexity of individual cases, fed by the lack of adequate information on outcomes and appropriateness and the fear of lawsuit, encourages extensive use of many new tests and procedures.

Patients, bombarded with news of exciting new treatments and wonder drugs, sometimes expect medicine to perform miracles. Some new techniques do, indeed, seem miraculous, such as imaging parts of the body heretofore seen only through extensive surgery. New tests can uncover problems earlier than ever, and some new procedures are more effective than ever. Our high technology society has a propensity to develop costly new high technologies which consumers have learned to demand. But more and more studies raise serious questions whether high technology results in better outcomes of care. In addition, we seem to desire these advances more ardently than we want to pay for them. (4)

Reimbursement policies in place for a generation have also created an incentive to provide services that in turn increase costs. Physicians are paid for each clinical service rendered, thus creating an incentive to offer more services. New technologies constantly pouring into the market further fuel this incentive. Meanwhile, physicians are not rewarded adequately for thinking about and implementing better care for the patient at less cost.

The looming threat of malpractice suits provides another powerful incentive for physicians to conduct many tests and procedures, particularly in high risk specialty areas such as obstetrics and gynecology and neurosurgery. Every patient is a potential litigant whose care could be questioned by a judge who may ask, not whether the most appropriate care was rendered effectively and efficiently, but whether all available tests and procedures were done for the patient. The result is that physicians sometimes feel compelled to practice defensive medicine, to perform tests and procedures solely to avoid lawsuit. While defensive medicine may sometimes improve the quality of care, it also results in excessive use of services. The precise amount is unknown, but some studies indicate it may be substantial.

Other factors also contribute to dramatic increases in health care costs. The growing supply of physicians—now 2.2 for every 1,000 people and projected to reach 2.6 by the year 2000—is expected to continue to increase costs rather than decrease them. The nation also has too many acute hospital beds. Although the number of hospital beds has decreased in recent years—by 1.8 percent in 1984–85 and another 1 percent in 1985–86—the drop is small and not evenly distributed across areas. The national occupancy rate for hospitals was only 68.9 percent in 1987. Finally, organizations created to help hospitals and physicians be more efficient, while claiming to lower costs, may in fact introduce a new layer of cost to the health care system.

Government Efforts to Control Costs

Both Medicare and Medicaid have helped the elderly and the poor to meet their basic health care needs, but they are flawed and expensive programs. Both programs are growing rapidly and are seriously underfunded. They cost federal and state governments $88 billion in 1983 and $132 billion in 1988. The Medicare Hospital Insurance trust fund is expected to run out of money by 2005. One of the government's major cost containment efforts, the Medicare Prospective Payment System (PPS), was adopted in 1983. It had the immediate effect of slowing the increase in hospital costs; Medicare's hospital payments subsequently grew 8.2 percent a year, as opposed to 16.5 percent growth in each of the three previous years. After adjusting for inflation, PPS resulted in a 4.3 percent reduction in the real rate of increase in Medicare spending for inpatient hospital services. (5) Yet during 1983–86, Medicare's final payments for hospital services increased faster than had been predicted, so either the quantity or scope of services may have increased. (5)

In a second government effort to control costs, Medicare froze fees for participating physicians from July 1984 to May 1986 and, until the end of December 1986, for nonparticipating physicians. (A participating physician is one who agreed to accept Medicare's designated payment, including the patient's 20 percent copayment, as payment in full for services rendered.) Yet during this period, expenditures for all physician services increased 7.2 percent, and Medicare's expenditures for physician services increased 9.1 percent, suggesting there may have been an increase in procedures and office visits to compensate for lost revenues from the freeze on fees.[2] After the freeze was lifted, physician fees under Medicare in 1986 began increasing at the same rate as all physician fees, 11.1 percent, or ten times faster than the overall inflation rate in that year (5), which had been depressed by the collapse of oil prices.

Today, cost control measures include the areas of physician payment and other outpatient services. The Congress, with advice forthcoming from the Health Care Financing Administration (HCFA) and the Physician Payment Review Commission (PPRC), is now considering whether to implement for Medicare the results of a Harvard University study conducted by a team led by Dr. Hsiao. This study developed a "relative value scale" (RVS) for physician fees based on the costs of providing various services. If adopted for payment, it would place greater value on primary care and less on tertiary care than the current system. Dr. William Roper, Administrator of HCFA, has pointed out that while such a system might be desirable and might reduce price inequities, it probably would not significantly reduce the total cost of Medicare's payments to physicians. (6) To control total payments, the volume and intensity of services need to be controlled, or total expenditures need to be capped.

Despite 15 years of active public and private efforts to cut costs, U.S. health care expenditures have quadrupled and are still rising at rates much higher than the Consumer Price Index (CPI). Expenditures for health care increased 6.3 percent in 1986 (after adjusting for population growth and overall inflation), while the CPI rose 2.5 percent that year. And the rate of increase in health care spending was over ll percent just two years later, when general inflation was close to 4.5 percent. These increases suggest that providers are using more technology, personnel, and services per capita. (5)

Private Efforts to Control Costs

In the private sector, cost containment has become a rallying cry in recent years. Concern about containing costs grew out of the explosive increase in company-paid health insurance for workers and their families during the labor-scare postwar years when companies lured employees with attractive benefit packages. At first the cost of those benefits could be passed on in full to the consumer, since U.S. dominance of world markets enabled business to set world prices for their products.

---

[2]For a more detailed explanation of research findings, see Dr. Janet Mitchell, President of the Center for Health Economics Research, testimony before the Physician Payment Review Commission, Washington, D.C., July 14, 1988.

But the U.S. economic position has changed. First, many of the early postwar employees have begun to retire, creating a large number of beneficiaries in an age group in need of substantial health care. Also, U.S. companies are no longer unilaterally able to set the price of their products. They compete with foreign companies with a less burdensome benefit structure. Increasingly challenged by international competition, U.S. companies are taking a close look at their costs across the board.

Consider the situation of General Motors (GM). While GM currently employs about 520,000 workers in the U.S., it provides coverage for over 2 million people, almost 1 percent of the entire U.S. population. GM therefore covers more retirees (over 300,000) and family members than it does employees. The company's bill for its generous health care benefits totalled $2.9 billion in 1987, an increase of over 20 percent, or $600 million, over the previous year, despite a decline in the number of active workers. Put another way, GM's health care bill absorbed the revenue from the sale of the equivalent of 270,000 of its cars. (7)

Some of the reasons for the increase in GM's costs are similar to those for industry as a whole. Like many segments of the manufacturing sector, the ratio of active workers to retirees is declining and now stands at fewer than two workers for every retiree. Second, the average age of the manufacturing sector's work force is increasing, and older people use more health services than younger workers. About 90 percent of the retiree population receives health care on a fee-for-service basis; such coverage incorporates few controls on use and is more expensive than increasingly popular managed care systems.

Like many other large corporations, GM offers its employees and their families a rich benefit package through an Informed Choice Plan that gives enrollees the choice of traditional fee-for-service, Preferred Provider Organizations (PPOs), or Health Maintenance Organizations (HMOs). Recent studies show higher rates of inpatient services for GM-covered patients than for the population as a whole. The steps GM is taking to change this pattern reflect steps being taken by industry as a whole. First, the company has developed an information system to study health claims data and pinpoint marked variations in care that merit further analysis. Secondly, GM has implemented programs that reflect national trends—programs that facilitate case management, control substance abuse, and encourage the use of generic and mail order prescription drugs, hospital admission pre-determination, and limits on approval for some new technologies. GM also instituted copayments and deductibles for salaried employees.

These steps have met with only moderate success, as signified by the cost increase GM experienced from 1986 to 1987. Private industry as a whole has had a similar experience. As a result, companies are considering new methods of selecting providers with good practice patterns. After identifying such providers, employers hope to trade volume for price through selective contracting, offering providers a large number of patients in return for a discount on the price of services and control of utilization. For example, GM is currently examining its utilization data with the goal of building a system to identify good providers of care—defined by GM as those who do not perform a high level of unnecessary services—and reward them with a larger share of GM's business. In some areas, groups of smaller companies are considering joining together to bargain with providers.

Private efforts have also been targeted to reducing their hospital costs. Aided by the government's PPS system, the efforts of private insurers appeared to have been successful in 1983–86 in controlling hospital costs, but the price for that success may have been higher costs than might otherwise have occurred in other areas, such as administrative costs and outpatient care. During those years, the rate of increase in hospital charges has been cut in half, while the rate of increase in physicians' fees and administrative costs has not been reduced as dramatically.[3] (8)

The emphasis on controlling hospital costs has led to a shift from inpatient care to outpatient services. For example, Coopers and Lybrand has documented a 70 percent increase in outpatient surgery since 1983. Yet, outpatient surgery for cataract removal costs an average of $4000, while the same surgery performed in a hospital runs about half that amount. According to HCFA, "outpatient reimbursement grew more rapidly than reimbursements for any other source" from 1967 to 1983. (8) These expenditures are expected to grow at an average annual rate of 14.5 percent, compared with the expected average annual growth rate of 7.3 percent for inpatient care. (9)

During the 1980s, private employers also turned to new mechanisms for providing care as a way to hold down costs. They encouraged employees to join HMOs, PPOs, and prepaid health plans. Many companies became self-insured to manage their own costs. Many employers have increased copayments and deductibles, both as a way to reduce their costs and to show the employee the actual cost of his or her health care, a reality from which many had been protected by extensive employer-provided health insurance. Another widespread phenomenon

---

[3]Hospital costs increased 6.2 percent as opposed to 15 percent for the preceding three years. Physician fees increased at an annual rate of 9.8 percent and the cost of administration jumped 15 percent, areas that had increased in the preceding three years by 12.5 and 21 percent, respectively. (8)

has been the requirement of second opinions as a way to reduce expensive procedures, such as major surgery.

Today, then, both government and large employers are developing plans to hold down cost increases. Change has already come in the areas of what services would be covered and the number and type of providers supported through HMOs and PPOs. Some employers are increasing copayments and deductibles and instituting cost-sharing for premiums. The large payers are clearly no longer willing to reimburse medical expenses without question. Their earlier attitude of not questioning charges and payments shielded physicians and patients alike from making economic considerations a part of their decisions and thus may have fueled increases in the volume of procedures and the cost of care. It is now clear that to control costs, the volume and intensity of services must be controlled, or failing that, total expenditures need to be capped.

Public Attitudes About Health Care and Costs

Despite the large cost increases in health care costs in recent years, opinion polls until recently consistently showed that Americans, while highly critical of some aspects of the health care system, were largely satisfied with their own care. The majority of Americans (54 percent in 1986) believed the U.S. spent too little on health care, and an even larger percentage (63 percent) wanted to make health care more available to those without it. Their concern with costs was not over the nation's costs but over rising costs to the individual. A sizable majority (70 percent) of the public believed these cost increases are not justified because the quality of care had not increased. Many people attributed increased costs to "too great a desire for profits among health care providers."

These polls showed that four options attracted public support for cost control: freezing hospital and physician fees, regionalizing big-ticket technologies, reducing inefficiencies in the service system (including unnecessary tests and hospital stays), and limiting care for the poor. The public declared a preference for more and better health care, including catastrophic care, long-term care, and high-technology medicine. And in 1987, the polls showed Americans continue to support equal access to health care for all Americans without concern for ability to pay but were willing to pay the taxes necessary. Thus, the public held conflicting views on cost control and access to care. (10)

A new poll conducted in 1988 by Louis Harris and Associates, in conjunction with the Harvard School of Public Health, found that a dramatic shift has recently taken place in American attitudes toward their health care system. Harris found that today "A striking 89 percent of Americans see the U.S. health-care system as requiring fundamental change in its direction and structure. Only 10 percent see their health-care arrangements as working reasonably well." (11) Only 54 percent of Americans told Harris they were very satisfied with their last physician encounter, while only 57 percent who were hospitalized in the last year said they were very satisfied with their hospital stay. The belief in the necessity of a fundamental shift in the direction of U.S. health-care policy is so strong, Harris reported, that "the majority of Americans say they would prefer a system like the Canadian health-care system to the one they currently have." (12)

DIMINISHING ACCESS FOR MILLIONS

The present patchwork system of health care does not provide effective and needed care to millions of Americans. This country has always had many people without health insurance and thus with often inadequate care. Throughout the 1970s, for example, there were about 25 million Americans without health insurance. (13) By the early 1980s that number had grown to about 37 million; their lack of insurance makes it more difficult for them to receive care.

In the seventies, as through much of our history, physicians and hospitals were expected to deliver free care to the uninsured, paid for by increasing the charges for those covered by insurance or otherwise able to pay. With the current financial picture dramatically changed and third-party payers resisting cost shifting and insisting on holding down specific charges on their bills, it has become much more difficult for physicians and hospitals to continue the traditional practice of shifting the costs of uncompensated care onto paying patients.

Most of the uninsured, between 70 and 75 percent, either work or are the dependents of workers. But they usually work in jobs where health insurance is not offered; 90 percent of uninsured workers are not offered health insurance by their employers, according to one estimate. (14) Sometimes health insurance is offered only to the employee and not his or her dependents. Many workers in these categories cannot afford private insurance or choose not to take it because of their low wages. Roughly one-third of the working uninsured falls below the federal poverty line, another one-third earns between 100 percent and 200 percent of the poverty level, and another third earns more.

Problems with Medicaid

The Medicaid program, originally designed to be the nation's safety net, now covers less than one-half of those in need. Low levels of coverage in some states—combined with the fact that the levels have often not kept pace with inflation—mean that Medicaid coverage of the poor and near poor has dropped from 60 to 46 percent since the program began in 1965. (15) Only one of every three poor women of childbearing age is covered by Medicaid, and lack of prenatal and infant care contributes to the high infant mortality rate in this country: eleven deaths per 1,000 babies born, which ranks us nineteenth among industrial nations. Medicaid devotes as little as 25 percent of its expenditures to low-income families with children, although they make up 70 percent of the program's recipient population. Because no other program finances long-term care, almost half of Medicaid expenditures go to these needs, primarily for the elderly.

Families of the "working poor" are ineligible for Medicaid coverage in many states. The result is that almost one-third of the uninsured, 11.2 million, are children. Each state's Medicaid eligibility level is tied to eligibility under Aid to Families with Dependent Children (AFDC). This has resulted in wide variations between states. In Massachusetts, a family of four must have a monthly income level below $891 to quality; in Alabama, the ceiling for a family of three is only $118 a month.

The uninsured, disproportionately minorities and the poor, have few choices when they do need medical care. The emergency room of the nearest hospital often becomes their family physician. In 1986, a Robert Wood Johnson Foundation survey found that one million people were denied care for financial reasons; 80 percent of these people were black, Hispanic, uninsured, or poor. The same survey found that almost 8 million people with chronic or serious illness did not seek care when it was needed, and another nearly 15 million Americans encountered barriers to care for economic reasons. (16) Another Robert Wood Johnson Foundation study conducted in the District of Columbia in 1988 found that the uninsured did not seek treatment until their condition was far more serious than that of the insured when they sought access to the system.

Failure to seek preventive or early care can both compound problems and ultimately raise costs. Those who do seek care for serious conditions, usually in the hospital, incur expensive unpaid bills that must be absorbed by the hospital and attending physicians. The result is uninsured, often minority, patients being "dumped"—denied emergency services or shifted from hospital to hospital—as the number of indigents has grown and providers have been increasingly unable to bill others for caring for the uninsured.

While Medicare and Medicaid provide essential services for the elderly and the poor, they have also led to the eclipse of the traditional system of hospitals and physicians providing free care to those who could not pay. The spirit of philanthropy, although an incomplete and sometimes undignified way to provide care, is now a much more limited phenomenon. The result has been less access to the system for those who fall through the cracks of the government's two major health care programs.

Even the beneficiaries of public programs are not always assured ready access to essential health care services. The disparity between the actual cost of services and Medicaid's reimbursement rate forces many physicians and hospitals to limit the number of Medicaid recipients they will serve. Twenty-five percent of all office-based physicians do not accept any Medicaid patients. (17) This rate is much higher for some specialties, especially obstetrics and gynecology, due also in part to high rates of litigation.

Problems with Medicare and Long-Term Care

Gaps in government programs mean that half the total cost of health care for the aged is paid for directly by the elderly person or the family. (18) So Medicare does not sufficiently ensure access to all necessary health care services for the elderly, who sometimes have high out-of-pocket expenses resulting from sizable copayment requirements in some covered services, and gaps in coverage for others such as prescription drugs and custodial nursing home care. This problem was ameliorated, but not solved, by the enactment of catastrophic coverage under Medicare last year. Catastrophic coverage could, in fact, further accelerate rising costs.

Changes in Medicare reimbursement policies added other problems for the elderly. For example, Medicare implemented a method of fixed advance payment to hospitals based on diagnosis-related groups (DRGs). This policy, directed at saving hospitalization costs, did not take into account the resulting shift of responsibility and expense to non-hospital sources of care. In many communities these nonhospital sources were not equipped to accept the influx of patients. Many families, home-health agencies, nursing homes, and other providers of care were overwhelmed.

Inpatient services were converted into outpatient services to cut hospital costs. Medicare hospital expenses became Part B outpatient expenses. Part A saved but Part B spent. Since Part B is funded from general revenues (in contrast to payroll taxes underpinning Part A), the DRG strategy added to the federal deficit and increased political pressures to curtail Part B spending. The DRG strategy also exposed individual patients and families to Part B copayments and to expenses not covered by Medicare, particularly care in the home.

In the face of substantial out-of-pocket expenses, poor and non-poor elderly who rely on Medicare are less likely to use physician services, drugs, and hospital services than those who can afford supplemental private coverage or are eligible for Medicaid.

Population trends and rising costs will cause access problems to worsen unless dramatic steps are taken. The elderly are a rapidly growing part of the population, their numbers soaring from 25.5 million in 1980 to 30.3 million in 1988. The very elderly over 85, many of whom are the "frail elderly," are growing at an even faster rate: their number of 2.24 million in 1980 is expected to more than double to 4.92 million by the year 2000.

In the twenty-first century, this issue will loom even larger. The U.S. elderly population will double by the year 2025, when one in five Americans will be over 65. Simultaneously, we will have three times as many people, or 6.2 million, over 80. Since illness and disability rates accelerate after age 75, these population trends will demand commitments to geriatrics-oriented systems of service. Specifically, acute-care and long-term care services must be carefully coordinated: the hospital, nursing home, home-care agency, and private physician cannot function in isolation. Linkages between health and social services are also essential, and the integration must be suitably financed. The goal is to accommodate frail and disabled individuals systematically, rather than in the existing fragmented way.

Action Needed on Long-Term Care

Current payment policies ignore the continuum of services needed by frail and disabled individuals. As we move into the twenty-first century, integrating health services will be crucial. For example, 300,000 patients move annually between hospital and nursing home, reflecting shifting needs for acute care and long-term care. Costs are paid differently in these categories of service and this, in itself, creates barriers to cooperation and, therefore, efficient and effective care.

The Commission believes in the concept of service integration and the necessary underlying financial integration. Barriers at either or both levels interfere with appropriate care. Acute care for the elderly is the domain of Medicare. Long-term care is covered largely by individuals and families out-of-pocket or by Medicaid. Private insurance for long-term care has been held up as the solution of the future, promising relief to Medicaid programs and families. Unfortunately, private insurance has had a limited presence in this area and, therefore, has not led the way to the integration of acute/long-term care and health and social services that is needed for effective geriatric care, especially for the very old.

Custodial long-term care is the most critical need for the elderly, yet Medicare meets few of these needs. The elderly must impoverish themselves down to the AFDC levels acceptable in their state in order to qualify for Medicaid, which does provide long-term care coverage. Younger adults and children with chronic conditions and in need of long-term care also have nowhere to turn for care they can afford.

In fact, by the year 2000, an estimated 40 percent of those in need of long-term care will be under 65. The Commission is concerned about the extent of health insurance for this group, because many of the new jobs being generated by the economy are in service industries, where health insurance has traditionally been less extensive than in the manufacturing sector. Trends toward part-time and temporary employment also contribute to the growth in the numbers of uninsured and their dependents. There is clearly a need for an intergenerational perspective in framing strategies to meet population needs.

The Commission did not specifically address long-term care, which has been studied by a number of Commissioners, some of whom, such as Alice Rivlin of Brookings, have made important proposals in this area. The Commission believes the urgent problems in this area should be addressed through the public-private partnership, shared responsibility approach which the Commission proposes for the overall health system. The Commission applauds recent action by the Congress to establish a Commission on Long-Term Care. When completed, recommendations from this study should be integrated into ours so a continuum of efficient care can be achieved.

PROBLEMS IN THE APPROPRIATENESS, EFFECTIVENESS, AND QUALITY OF CARE

Serious problems exist in the quality and appropriateness of much of the medical care being rendered. A major reason for this is the high degree of uncertainty pervading medical practice. The Commission was surprised to find uncertainty emerging, in study after study in recent years, as an issue in every area of medicine. It has become clear to the Commission over the past two years that uncertainty in medical practice was a problem, not just in a few specialties, but that it was generic to the practice of medicine. Due in part to the fact that medicine is an art as well as a science, doctors will always face uncertainty, but the Commission believes that the current level of uncertainty can and must be decreased.

Uncertainty in medicine is evidenced by the wide variations in medical practice reported between regions, cities, and even hospitals in the same city. In pioneering work by Dr. John Wennberg, of the Dartmouth Medical School, the state of Maine was studied. Maine was chosen for variation studies because it was one of the first states to mandate the collection of total hospital discharge data. Analysis of Maine data reveals marked variation in hospitalizations for many procedures, sometimes five or ten times more hospitalizations for certain procedures in some areas than in others. For example, hospital admissions for pneumonia in different communities in Maine varied by a factor of five for adults and a factor of more than ten for children. Studies by the Maine Medical Assessment Program have determined that the principal reason is uncertainty among doctors as to the best treatment. (19)

Studies in other states reveal similar high variations in practice patterns between communities. Dr. John Wennberg compared hospital admissions among residents of Boston and New Haven, two populations very similar in characteristics that predict the demand for care. His team found that expenditures in hospitals were twice as much per city resident in Boston as in New Haven. While Boston and New Haven were found to have the same overall rates of surgery, rates for individual operations varied substantially. For example, there were more than twice as many carotid endarterectomies in Boston as in New Haven, while there were twice as many coronary artery bypass operations in New Haven as in Boston. Yet, the incidence of the underlying illnesses appears quite similar, based on rates of hospitalization for heart attack and stroke in both cities. The incidence of hysterectomies is substantially higher in New Haven, while knee and hip replacements are more frequent in Boston. There appeared to be no health or socioeconomic reasons for such discrepancies. (20)

The differences in hospitalization costs were largely explained by the remarkably higher rate of admission for a variety of commonplace medical conditions such as back pain, gastrointestinal conditions, diabetes, and pulmonary conditions. If the rate of use of hospitals beds among residents of Boston were the same as among the New Havenites, Boston area hospitals would need 525 fewer beds.

As early as the 1930s, differences such as these have been ascribed to "medical opinion" or practice style. The practice style of a physician may result from a number of factors—his or her formal training, experiences while in practice, and postgraduate education. The important question is why do practice styles differ so much? The underlying reason, it turns out, is lack of valid scientific evidence about the effects on patients of the various treatment theories that are behind the differences in practice styles. In other words, the basic problem is an inadequate scientific base for clinical decisionmaking, traceable to the lack of attention we as a society have paid to evaluating medical care outcomes, particularly with treatments other than drugs.

The treatment of threatened strokes due to narrowing of the arteries in the neck provides an example. While the use of aspirin compared to no treatment at all has been shown by scientific study to be effective in preventing stroke, no adequate comparisons have been made of the effectiveness of aspirin compared to the operative approach (carotid endarterectomy), nor has that operation been compared to no treatment at all. The quite natural result is confusion and disagreement among physicians concerning which approach is best because of unresolved uncertainty about when carotid endarterectomy is the correct treatment.

Uncertainty is not inevitable. In Maine, practicing physicians together with researchers at Dartmouth, Harvard, and the University of Massachusetts undertook a study to examine the practice style for variation in prostatectomy rates among Maine communities. The differences in medical opinion were traced to different theories urologists held about the outcomes for patients with obstruction of the urinary tract due to non-cancerous growth of the prostate. Some physicians believed in the "preventive theory of surgery"—they recommended that patients be operated on early in the course of the condition because they believed the operation resulted in an increased life expectancy. Others believed that for most patients the operation was useful for a different reason: it made patients feel better by reducing their symptoms.

Using several strategies for examining the difference in theory, the researchers were able to show that for most patients the operation does not increase life expectancy. They were also able to obtain much more precise estimates for symptom reduction and complication rates than had been previously available in the medical literature. Perhaps most important, the research documented the importance of patient preference in the choice of treatment, showing that some surgical patients, even some with severe symptoms, were not bothered very much by their symptoms before they had their operation.

The Maine outcome study thus leads to the conclusion that differences in practice style underlying the variation in rates were due to an inappropriate belief on the part of some physicians in the preventive theory of surgery and failure to take the preferences of some patients into account in recommending surgery.

Research results of such studies, even those with excellent evaluations, have too often been poorly disseminated. The inadequate information base has led to decisions of diagnosis and treatment practices that are often confused, contradictory, or even contrary to what evidence does exist.

When physicians do learn about carefully conducted studies with significant results, their practice patterns do change. Once urologists in

Maine were told the results of the study, the number of prostatectomies dropped by 15 percent. (20)

Studies conducted at the RAND Corporation have considered whether certain major, expensive procedures were appropriate. The physician panels looking at them have found rates of inappropriate care for four major procedures that ranged from 14 to 32 percent: 14 percent for coronary artery bypass surgery (with 30 percent equivocal), (21) 17 percent for upper GI tract endoscopy (11 percent equivocal), 17 percent for coronary angiography (9 percent equivocal), and 32 percent for carotid endarterectomy (32 percent equivocal). (22) Such inappropriate care may result in a great deal of unnecessary harm.

These and other similar studies have focused attention on these issues; investment in analysis of them remains seriously deficient. In 1986, the nation spent $475 billion on health care, but only $8.2 billion on health-related research. Most of that was basic research; only a few million dollars (less than .001 percent of our total health expenditures) went to outcomes research, aimed at assessing the efficacy of our medical care. Studies have been funded by private foundations and the federal government at places like RAND, the Joint Commission on the Accreditation of Healthcare Organizations, Duke University, Dartmouth University, and the Institute of Medicine. HCFA and the National Center for Health Services Research provide the bulk of federal funds for health services research. Despite limited funding, some foundations and private specialty organizations, such as the American Medical Association, the Blue Cross/Blue Shield Association, and the American College of Physicians, among others, have sponsored the development of information for evaluating specific practices.

Many of these groups have conducted important work, but the results are just one more piece in a patchwork of inadequate outcome information provided the medical profession. It is not that individual practitioners willfully ignore the latest clinical information, but rather that the complex scientific, legal, fiscal and social environments give conflicting signals. The lack of an effective information system for physicians, particularly those outside the major teaching centers, contributes to this problem. Therefore, even where practice policies have been carefully thought out and agreed upon by experts, they may not be utilized or may be improperly utilized by individual practitioners.

Even when technologies are known to be appropriate, wide variations exist in how competently and effectively they are applied. For example, outcomes for surgical procedures are often better in hospitals where more of those operations are performed. This information raises difficult policy questions for those concerned with providing high quality care to all who need it: Should those operations be limited, via regulation or payment policies, to certain hospitals? And how would such limitations affect access to those procedures?

In testimony before the Commission and in an article published recently in the *New England Journal of Medicine*, Dr. Donald Berwick of Harvard points out the problems which currently exist with health care quality assurance systems. Human error is inevitable in a process as complex as health care in which physicians must deal with many complex diseases. It is therefore mandatory to have in place adequate quality control and assurance systems. Unfortunately, health care has remained largely insulated from modern methods of quality control. Inspection remains the main form of quality assurance and there is little evidence of appreciation of the importance of designing quality into the front end of our services.

The sad fact is that in regard to inpatient care, our quality control systems are at best rudimentary. Hospitals have traditionally focused only on how care is delivered: they have just begun to measure the impact of that care on patient outcomes. Quality control systems are even less developed in the office ambulatory setting and nursing home where more and more care is being delivered. Most errors and quality problems in health care are due to faulty systems design or inadequate information and not to willful neglect. (23) Yet, out of a $500 billion annual health care expenditure, we have invested virtually nothing in the tools for designing quality into our services. We have invested pitifully inadequate amounts into determining whether much of what we are doing is done well, or worth doing in the first place, or in developing guidelines for care which can be monitored.

If hospitals and ambulatory practices are often ill-equipped to do first-rate assessments, patients are even further behind in their ability to make informed choices and decisions about their care. Examples abound of diagnostic tests whose primary purpose is to reassure the patient or the doctor that the original treatment choice was correct. Such tests do not change the actual course of patient management, but they do have benefits, albeit difficult ones to quantify. We must learn better how to relate these benefits to their costs, while allowing for individual preferences. When the course of treatment includes choices, the patient, like the physician should be guided by solid assessments of the appropriateness and effectiveness of the different options.

One of the problems in the system has clearly been that patients have been ill-equipped and perhaps not adequately motivated to take strong personal responsibility for their own health care. They have certainly not clearly understood the costs and benefits of proposed tests and treatments. They have not asked good questions. While many have improved their lifestyles, others refuse to do so in the face of persistent medical advice on the importance of healthy lifestyles.

The prevailing pattern in health care is persistent intervention in the face of persistent uncertainty. One physician recently described in the *Journal of the American Medical Association* the "cascades of cardiology." He wrote of processes that, once started, are hard to stop. "One test leads to another and then another, with too little pause to think in between." A patient with unusual chest pain receives an exercise test that shows suspicious changes, leading to an isotope study resulting in suggestive defects in a shadowy image, thus leading to an arteriogram showing some coronary artery disease, "and so on down the cascade" of tests and procedures. The physician ordering each procedure may also perform and be paid for each one, interpret the results, and order still more tests. That is not to say, according to the author, that these procedures are all done for the financial gain of the physician or institution, but he believes the temptation is there. (24) Many observers are concluding that there are perverse incentives built deep into the structure of our health care system.

CONCLUSION

In summary, what we find is a system under great stress with serious cost, access, and quality problems which are inextricably intertwined. Costs are rising rapidly and access is a problems for many Americans, including 11 million children. An article in the *Journal of the American Medical Association* by Dr. Marcia Angell, the deputy editor of the *New England Journal of Medicine*, addressed the question: Is more medical care better? She concludes that "far from being beneficial, much of the medical care in this country is unnecessary, is of no demonstrated value to those who receive it, and some of it is harmful." (25)

These critical problems in the cost, appropriateness, quality, and access to health care in America present a clear and compelling case for change. These problems are interrelated and systemic. They will require comprehensive, integrated solutions. Piecemeal approaches will not work. We face a complex of problems that we now realize can be effectively solved only in relation to one another. For example, until we come to agreement on the definition of quality and appropriate care, it will be difficult to know what is worth providing access to and what is worth paying for. Change in one area forces change, often unintended, in another area, as this country has painfully learned. To mitigate further error and the compounding of already serious problems, the Commission proposes an orderly progression of systemwide changes over the coming years.

As part of its deliberations, the Commission explored the possibility of calling for short-term action on cost control while steps were being taken to improve access and quality of care and to put in place a system that is inherently more efficient and more cost-sensitive. The rationale for such a move was clear: by the time systemic improvements in the health care system can be put in place in several years, costs will have increased several hundred billion dollars. Yet it was also clear that one of the lessons we have learned from the changes attempted over the past decades in health care is that a cutback in one area may mean increases in another. A freeze on fees, for example, could just mean an increase in volume, in the number of procedures being done. The result might not be to decrease overall costs at all. Exploration of this area only heightened the Commission's resolve to call for broad change in the American health care system.

The Commission has deliberated long and hard on these problems; this report presents its recommendations for action to redesign our health care system so that it can make available to all quality health care at a reasonable cost.

REFERENCES

1. Relman, A., "Assessment and Accountability: The Third Revolution," *NEJM*, 319(18):1220–1222, November 3, 1988.
2. Berry, J., *Financier Magazine*, December 1988, p. 7.
3. Crenshaw, A., *Washington Post*, January 8, 1989.
4. Blendon, R., "The Public's View of the Future of Health Care," *JAMA* 259(24):3587–3593, June 24, 1988.
5. Anderson, G., and Erickson, J., "National Medical Spending," *Health Affairs* 6(3):96–104, Fall 1987.
6. Roper, W., "Perspectives on Physician-Payment Reform: The Resource-Based Relative-Value Scale in Context," *NEJM* 319(13):865–867, September 29, 1988.
7. Beach Hall, statement to National Leadership Commission on Health Care, March 1988.
8. Department of Health and Human Services, Health Care Financing Administration, *Health Care Financing Review: Program Statistics, Medicare and Medicaid Databook, 1986*, Publication 03247, September 1987, pp. 21–29.
9. "Projection of Health Care Spending to 1990," *Health Care Financing Review* 7(3):1–35, Spring 1986, p. 2.
10. Blendon, R., "The Public's View of the Future of Health Care," *JAMA* 259(24):3587–3593, June 24, 1988.
11. Blendon, R., "Three Systems: A Comparative Survey," *Health Management Quarterly* 11(1):2–10, First Quarter 1989, p. 3.
12. Blendon, R., "Three Systems: A Comparative Survey," *Health Management Quarterly* ll(1):2–10, First Quarter l989, pp. 4–5.
13. Congressional Budget Office, "Profile of Health Care Coverage: The Haves and Have-Nots," background paper, March 1979.
14. Wilensky, G., "Solving Uncompensated Hospital Care," in M.B. Sulvetta and K. Swartz, *The Uninsured and Uncompensated Care: A Chartbook*, National

Health Policy Forum, George Washington University, Washington, DC, June 1986.

15. Blendon, R., et al., "Uncompensated Care by Hospitals or Public Insurance for the Poor: Does it Make A Difference?" *NEJM* 314(18):1160–1163, May 1, 1986.
16. *SPECIAL REPORT, Access to Health Care in the United States: Results of a 1986 Survey*, November 2, 1987, The Robert Wood Johnson Foundation.
17. "Medicaid Mill: Fact or Fiction," *Health Care Financing Review* 2(1):37–49, Summer 1980.
18. Health Care Financing Administration, Annual Report, 1987.
19. Statement by Keller, R., before the U.S. Senate Committee on Finance, Subcommittee on Health, July 11, 1988.
20. Wennberg, J., "The Medical Care Outcome Problem: An Agenda for Action," paper prepared for the National Leadership Commission on Health Care, May 1987.
21. Winslow, C., Kosecoff, J., et al., "The Appropriateness of Performing Coronary Artery Bypass Surgery," *JAMA* 260(4):505–509, July 22/29, 1988.
22. Chassin, M., Kosecoff, J., et al., "Does Inappropriate Use Explain Geographic Variations in the Use of Health Care Services?" *JAMA* 258(18):2533–2537, November 13, 1987.
23. Berwick, D., "Continuous Improvement as an Ideal in Health Care," *NEJM* 320(1):53–56, January 5, 1989.
24. James, T., "Cascades, Collusions, and Conflicts in Cardiology," *JAMA* 259(16):2454–2455, April 22/29, 1988.
25. Angell, M., "Cost Containment and the Physician," *JAMA* 254(9):1203–1207, September 6, 1985, p. 1204.

ADDENDA

The following paragraphs of Chapter One have been updated with information that has come to light since the NLC Report was originally published. Changes have been italicized. Roman numeral superscripts refer to new notes; online numbers refer to original notes.

Page 2, Paragraph 4:...In the *25* years since the passage of Medicare, national health care expenditures have increased more than tenfold—from $41.9 billion, or 5.9 percent of GNP to *$600* billion, or *11.5* percent of GNP.[i]

Page 3, Paragraphs 4 and 5:...Costs have increased tenfold in the last 25 years and continue to rise rapidly....In the year 2000, health care will consume 15 percent of GNP, and this country will spend *$5,550* on health care for every man, woman, and child.[ii] In *1988*, health care costs rose *10.4* percent to *$539.9 billion, or 11.1 percent of GNP*. Physician fees *increased 13.1 percent in 1988*.[iii]

We currently spend *an estimated $660 billion, or about 12 percent of our GNP* on health care, much more per capita than any other nation, and our cost escalation outstrips that of any other country.[iv]

Page 7, Paragraph 2:... Although the number of hospital beds has decreased in recent years—*from 1,267,000 beds in 1987 to 1,248,000 in 1988*—the drop is small and not evenly distributed across areas. The national occupancy rate for hospitals was only *69.2 percent in 1988.*[v]

Page 8, Paragraph 2:...The Congress, with advice from the Physician Payment Review Commission (PPRC) and the administration, *passed a law in 1989 adopting a fee schedule for Medicare. The new schedule will be based on resource costs, using in part a Harvard University study, conducted by a team led by Dr. Hsaio, which developed a "relative value scale" (RVS) for physician fees and also used geographic variables studied by HCFA. The new law places greater value on primary care and less on tertiary care than the current system. Dr. William Roper, former administrator of HCFA, has pointed out that while an RVS system alone* might be desirable and might reduce price inequities, it probably would not significantly reduce the total cost of Medicare's payments to physicians.(6) To control total payments, the volume and intensity of services need to be controlled, or total expenditures need to be capped. *The PPRC proposal, adopted in modified form in the new law, includes a version of expenditure targets called "volume performance standards."*[vi]

Despite 15 years of active public and private efforts to cut costs, U.S. health care *expenditures are still rising* at rates much higher than the Consumer Price Index (CPI). [*Delete:* Expenditures for health care...close to 4.5 percent.]

Page 13, Paragraph 1: half of Medicaid expenditures go to these needs, primarily for the elderly.[vii]

Page 14, Paragraph 3: *Delete:* "This problem was ameliorated. ...accelerate rising costs.

New References

i.   U.S. Department of Commerce, *U.S. Industrial Outlook 1990—Health Services,* 1990, p. 49-1.
ii.   "National Health Expenditures, 1986–2000," *Health Care Financing Review* 8 (4):18, Summer 1987.
iii. U.S. Department of Health and Human Services, Health Care Financing Administration, "National Health Expenditures, 1988," draft report, May 1990, pp. 1, 10.
iv.   U.S. Department of Commerce, *U.S. Industrial Outlook 1990—Health Services,* 1990, p. 49-6.
v.   American Hospital Association, *Hospital Statistics,* AHA, Chicago, 1989, p. 2.
vi.   Physician Payment Review Commission, "Physician Payment Reform: Summary of Provisions of H.R. 3299, Omnibus Budget Reconciliation Act of 1989," draft paper, December 11, 1989.
vii. U.S. Department of Health and Human Services, Health Care Financing Administration, "National Health Expenditures, 1988," draft report, May 1990, p. 23.

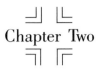

Chapter Two

Financing Access to the Health Care System—The Commission's Plan: A Shared Responsibility

Public-opinion polls indicate that Americans take a strongly egalitarian view toward health policy. In response to the question, "Should all Americans have access to the same level of quality in health care, regardless of ability to pay?" over 80 percent in a recent, nation-wide survey answered "yes" and fewer than eight percent said "no." (1)

These noble sentiments stand in stark contrast to current American health policy. The United States today is the only major industrialized country without a health insurance system that guarantees universal access to at least a basic package of health benefits. Some 37 million Americans now lack health insurance of any kind during at least some period of the year.

Whatever the reason for this disparity between professed ideals and actual practice, the problem of the uninsured must be addressed explicitly, lest the American health system develop unacceptable inequities. The Commission's extensive deliberations on this issue have led to the concrete policy recommendations set forth in this chapter.

The Commission began its deliberations by articulating basic principles that should guide a policy to bring the uninsured into the comprehensive health insurance system that covers the vast majority of Americans. These principles are presented in the next section, together with a discussion on the compromises among competing principles that must be made in building politically and economically viable policy recommendations.

The Commission recognized early on that the nation's un-willingness to strike such compromises among cherished principles has been the major stumbling block in the development of a policy that does justice to our professed ideals. In his highly perceptive "Allocating Health Resources," ethicist Daniel Callahan argues that uncertainties "over our national values are ultimately the source of our problem in fairly allocating health care," (2) a diagnosis also offered earlier by Com-mission member Uwe Reinhardt in his "Hard Choices in Health Care: A Matter of Ethics." (3)

Following the discussion of basic principles, this chapter presents the health insurance proposal developed by the Commission. It is a blend of two proposals widely discussed among health-policy analysts: a) mandating the individual's responsibility for obtaining adequate health insurance coverage, and b) encouraging employers to provide basic health insurance to all employed Americans, with the public sector assuming responsibility for the rest.

Basic Principles Underlying the Commission's Proposal to Provide Care for the Uninsured

Reflecting both their own and the general public's ethical beliefs, the Commissioners agreed that the American health system should live up to the fundamental

I. *Principle of Universal Access*:

There should be no financial barrier separating Americans in need of health care from access to basic care.

This principle implies simply that the probability of gaining physical relief, of recuperating to a given degree, or of surviving a given episode of illness or trauma ought not to be a function of the patient's financial resources.

It does not imply that every American should enjoy completely free (first dollar) access to needed health services. On the contrary, the Com-mission believes that patients should bear some of the cost of their care in the form of copayments, deductibles and coinsurance, up to an an-nual maximum that varies with income.[1] Such cost sharing encourages patients to understand bills submitted by providers and to become pru-dent purchasers of health care.

---

[1]See the section of this chapter entitled Cost Sharing for a complete discussion and related Commission recommendations pertaining to this issue.

The *Principle of Universal Access* also does not imply that health services will be available to all Americans on completely equal terms, regardless of ability to pay. For example, the principle is not violated if some Americans secure for themselves, with their own financial resources, completely free choice among providers of health care, while others with more modest means are required to obtain publicly or privately financed care from closed panels, such as health maintenance organizations (HMOs) or preferred provider organizations (PPOs). Nor is the *Principle of Universal Access* violated if some patients secure for themselves superior amenities—e.g., private rooms—not easily affordable by low-income patients.

The Commissioners next agreed that implementing the Principle of Universal Access should come at the expense of society at large and not simply by tacit reliance on the noblesse oblige of providers. That sentiment was expressed in the

II. *Principle of Fair Compensation*:

Every provider and practitioner of health services should be reasonably compensated for services rendered to patients.

The Compensation Principle establishes that the United States should not finance health care for indigent or underinsured patients through the current combination of uncompensated care and cost shifting to paying patients. The Commission rejects this system because it reduces uninsured, lower-income Americans to relying on sometimes unreliable charity care; it forces providers to act as the collector of hidden taxes in their effort to seek compensation for health care; and it shifts the cost of such care to other payers—be they individuals, private business or government—who can pay additional charges.

The Commission recognizes that, whatever its current failings, the American health system stands out as probably the world's most dynamic and innovative health system. Mindful of the need for continued innovation, the Commissioners agreed on the

III. *Principle of Clinical and Economic Freedom*:

To the maximum extent possible, without unduly compromising other important principles, public health policy ought to restore *clinical freedom* in rendering health services, and *economic freedom* in making arrangements to finance these services, within the context of effective countervailing market power from those who ultimately pay for health care in America.

Providing health care for Americans who cannot afford to pay for it inevitably requires the diversion of resources from those who can pay.

That diversion can be achieved by explicit taxation or it can be achieved through less visible forms of diversion, such as hidden cost-shifting among patients or mandating employers to provide health insurance to employees.

A strong case can be made for making the cost of helping the poor visible and explicit. But Americans appear to be ambivalent on this subject. On the one hand, they want health care distributed on a universal basis. On the other hand, they resist the explicit taxation required to do so. A politically viable strategy toward the goal of universal access must spread the explicit cost of providing this care as widely as possible, relying on a system of multiple-source financing. Such a strategy is thus based on

IV. *The Principle of Shared Responsibility*:

Financial responsibility for the provision of health care for those too poor to afford it should be shared by government, individuals and employers.

The concept of a shared responsibility is central to this report, reflecting both the democratic principles of our society and the ad hoc sharing of costs that already exists in our health care system. A social contract must be developed that apportions the cost of providing health care to low-income Americans fairly among middle- and upper-income Americans.

This shared responsibility includes a central role for the individual patient. To describe that role, the Commission agreed, after lengthy deliberation, on:

V. *The Principle of Individual Responsibility*:

To help achieve the goal of universal access to health care, the individual has a duty to have adequate health insurance coverage at all times for him- or herself and for his or her dependent children.

The Commission notes the highly uneven incidence of annual health expenditures between individuals. As a general rule, only about 10 percent of the population in any given year accounts for 80 percent of total national health outlays, which implies that most health expenditures are incurred by severely ill patients with high health-care bills. An uninsured severely ill person is likely to saddle others with a sizable bill.

Uninsured people who benefit from the advanced technology of America's health care system, and may even owe their lives to it, ought not to be permitted to neglect to purchase health insurance they could actually afford. Estimates indicate that at least 20 percent to 30 percent of the currently uninsured could afford health insurance.

In considering whether responsibility for assuring all Americans access to health care should be a federal or a state and local responsibility, the Commission settled on a federal guarantee:

VI. *The Principle of Basic Benefits Guarantee*:

The design of a basic package of health-service benefits to which all Americans should have reliable access is ultimately a federal responsibility.

This principle does not exclude state and local governments from participating in a system designed to provide universal access. Nor does it imply rigid national uniformity in the design of benefit packages, compensation systems, and so on. But the principle does articulate the widely shared notions that 1) there ought to be a floor in health care beneath which no American will be permitted to sink, and 2) citizens in one state should take an interest in and bear some responsibility for what happens to suffering fellow Americans in other states. This principle is especially important in an age in which the economic fortunes of individual states can rise and fall rapidly with shifts in world trade. The Commission finds fundamentally flawed a health care system that exposes the level of care of American infants in Texas or Louisiana to the vagaries of oil-price policies hammered out overseas. With Medicaid payments set entirely by the states, our current system includes wide and fluctuating discrepancies. Finally, the Commission vigorously supports

VII. *The Principle of a Strong Doctor-Patient Relationship*:

Any health care system should foster the goal of protecting the integrity of the doctor-patient relationship.

No financing mechanism should in any way undermine the centrality of the doctor-patient relationship in the health care system. The integrity of that relationship should not be compromised by a system that encourages either the overuse or underuse of medical services.

A STRATEGY FOR PROVIDING UNIVERSAL ACCESS

General Description

On the basis of the fundamental principles set forth above, the Commission developed a strategy for providing all American citizens reliable access to needed health services on terms the individual can afford.[2]

---

[2]The Commission was ably assisted in designing its proposed strategy by the work done for the Commission by Lewin/ICF.

This system builds upon the American tradition of providing private health insurance through the workplace. It is designed to encourage continued extensive reliance on that approach without mandating that employers provide such coverage. Thus, the system preserves the pluralistic approach to health-care financing apparently preferred by Americans. Figures 1 and 2 display the changes in sources of funding under current policy and under the Commission's plan.

Figure 1: Source of Payments for Health Benefits Under Current Policy (in billions of 1988 dollars)

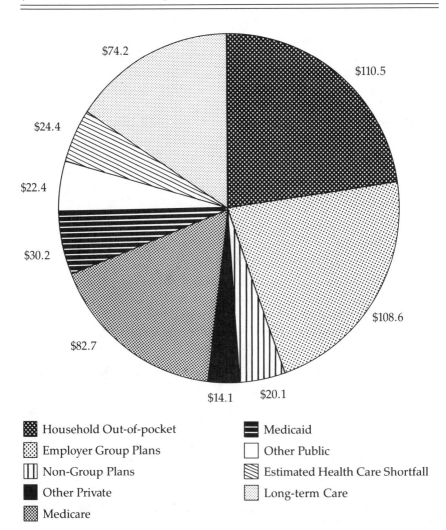

	Household Out-of-pocket		Medicaid
	Employer Group Plans		Other Public
	Non-Group Plans		Estimated Health Care Shortfall
	Other Private		Long-term Care
	Medicare		

The Commission's safety net system, designated by the Commission as the Universal Access (UNAC) program, would be administered at the state level by a cooperative effort involving all participants in the health care system. The federal government would provide guidelines for the program designed to provide all Americans with a basic level of services, regardless of location, but the program would not be centrally directed as is, for example, the Medicare program. There would be am-

Figure 2: Source of Payments for Health Benefits Under the Commission's Proposal (in billions of 1988 dollars)

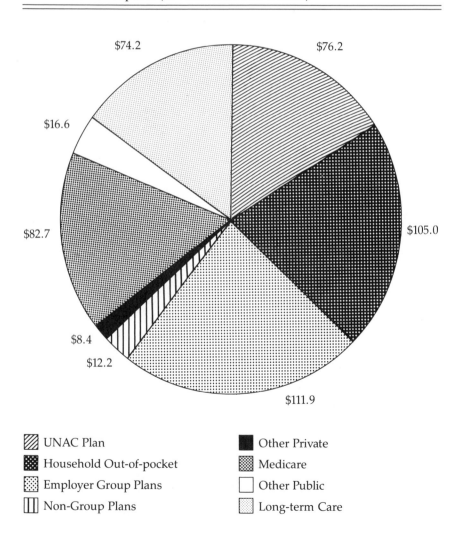

ple room for regional variations and local initiatives within the broad federal guidelines.

This proposal would extend health coverage to the 37 million Americans who now lack health insurance. All Americans would be responsible for having coverage for the national basic package of services. There are several ways they could obtain this coverage. Most Americans would probably continue to obtain privately-financed coverage as an employment benefit, with the employer contributing most or all of the money for the premium. Any American could also choose to purchase this coverage with personal funds or could supplement the employer-provided coverage with personal funds. Older Americans would continue to receive Medicare coverage. Everyone else would receive public coverage through the UNAC program. The Commission calls for a shared responsibility in financing UNAC. Although Americans with incomes below 150 percent of the poverty level[3] would have their premiums subsidized, they would be responsible for a small share of the costs of their care at the time of service.

The plan proposed by the Commission is designed to encourage everyone to have his or her own insurance coverage and to provide an incentive to employers to offer insurance coverage for a basic level of care. It is also designed to make the process fairer between employers, easing the burden on those companies who foot the health care bill for spouses who could be covered by their own employers, but choose not to be, usually because their plan is less generous.

The Commission's plan also uses strong incentives to encourage employers to offer coverage and to improve coverage under some existing plans. Employers who do not provide coverage to their employees would be required to pay a fee, known as the X_1 fee, which would finance the UNAC program to provide coverage to all uninsured workers and their dependents with incomes **above** 150 percent of the federal poverty level.

Employers who offer a health plan would be exempt from the X_1 fee if their plan

1. provides at least the basic national level of coverage,[4]
2. limits the employee contribution for that coverage to no more than 25 percent of the total premium, and
3. extends coverage to all full-time workers.[5]

---

[3]The federal poverty level for a family of four was about $11,170 in 1988.

[4]The Commission is not making a recommendation about what specific services should be in the national basic package of services, but is recommending a process for establishing and continually updating the package. See later in this chapter for more discussion.

[5]This provision applies to persons age 18 or older who work 25 or more hours per week.

Figure 3: Funding Mechanism for UNAC Program

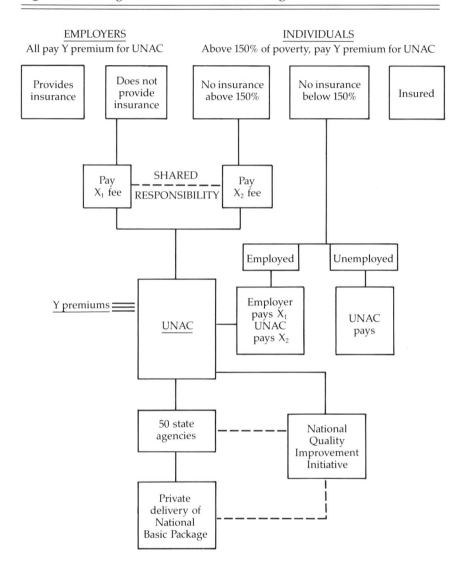

All employers would have a choice of providing coverage or paying the X_1 fee. We estimate that for firms whose average wages per employee exceed 250 percent of the poverty level for an individual, very few would select the coverage under UNAC. Employers who do not meet all three minimum standards would pay the full amount of the X_1 fee on all employees. The employer has the option of providing coverage to part-time workers who work less than 25 hours a week or to pay an X_1 fee for these workers, proportional to the hours worked. Special provisions are proposed for new businesses, small businesses, and new employees.

New Business: The X_1 fee for firms that do not provide health insurance would be reduced for firms in existence three years or less. The X_1 fee would be reduced by 60 percent for firms up to one year of age, 40 percent for firms up to two years of age, and 20 percent for firms up to 3 years of age. The full amount of the X_1 fee would be paid by firms over three years of age. The X_2 fee for employees (described below) of those businesses would remain the same.

Self-Employed Persons: Self-employed persons who do not have health insurance will be required to pay both the X_1 and the X_2 fees. To relieve the burden on this group of workers, the Commission proposes to reduce the combined fee by the same proportion that the social security FICA rate is reduced for self-employed persons (FICA for self-employed persons is about 86.7 percent of the combined employer/employee payment for wage and salary workers).

Small Firms: The X_1 fee for small firms (5 or fewer employees) that do not provide health insurance would be reduced by about 20 percent.

Part-Time Workers: The X_1 and X_2 fee rates would be paid only in proportion to the number of hours worked per week. For purposes of determining the amount of this fee, part-time workers are defined as persons working less than 35 hours per week.[6] For part-time workers, the X_1 and X_2 fee rates would be computed as the standard fee rates reduced by the proportion of the week they usually work. The purpose of this provision is to prevent the X_1 fee from discouraging employment of part-time workers and to lessen the X_2 fee burden on part-time workers who typically have low incomes.

In keeping with the dual Commission principles of a shared responsibility and individual responsibility, the plan also calls for a fee to

---

[6]Note that for purposes of scaling down the X_1 and X_2 fee rates for part-time workers, part-time worker in this instance is defined as an employee working less than 35 hours per week. This differs from the definition of part time used in determining whether an employer may cover the worker under the UNAC program, which is currently set at 25 hours per week.

be paid by individuals who do not have insurance.[7] This fee, known as the X_2 fee, would be levied on all uninsured individuals with incomes over 150 percent of the Federal poverty threshold. These individuals would, in turn, receive coverage under the UNAC program. The fee encourages individuals who have the opportunity to accept coverage from other sources to do so by exempting all covered persons from paying this fee.

The Commission plan includes an incentive designed to encourage a worker's own employer to pick up his or her coverage. Workers currently covered as dependents under their spouse's plan would have the option to either

1. accept coverage under their own employer's plan if offered, or

2. accept additional wraparound coverage from their spouse's employer, or

3. pay the X_2 fee and become covered with other workers under UNAC.

In addition, when both parents work, the plan calls for one of the employer's plans picking up the children. This choice would be made by the parents and their respective employers. These provisions are intended to encourage "inter-employer equity"[8] by shifting the cost of insuring some working dependents from their spouse's employer to their own employer. (4)

The UNAC program would also provide health insurance coverage to all current Medicaid participants, with the exception of those receiving long-term care, and all non-workers and all workers and their dependents with incomes **below** 150 percent of the federal poverty level. Medicaid would be restructured by UNAC[9] by establishing a basic level of services for everyone, thus eliminating the patchwork quilt of eligibility and coverage rules that comprise our current Medicaid system. States could supplement the UNAC package. Health benefits provided in the UNAC program would be financed with:

1. State and Federal revenues that would have been expended under the current Medicaid program, and

---

[7]This includes all uninsured individuals above 150 percent of the poverty level whether employed, unemployed, nonworking or retired who neither have subsidized coverage nor coverage purchased with their own funds.

[8]The Commission credits this term to Alain Enthoven.

[9]The Commission plan does not specifically address the question of long-term care. The Medicaid program would be restructured for preventive and acute care only and would be retained for long-term care.

2. An assessment on employers and individuals above 150 percent of the poverty level known as the Y health premium.

A small portion of the Y premium would be used to fund an additional investment in health services research, such as research on appropriateness of care or on the outcomes of competing treatments. (This is discussed in more detail later in this chapter, as well as in the chapter entitled "A National Quality Improvement Initiative.")

Summary of Estimates

As shown in Technical Appendix I, the most reasonable estimate is that about 67.9 million people will become covered under the UNAC pro-

Figure 4: National Health Expenditure and Universal Access

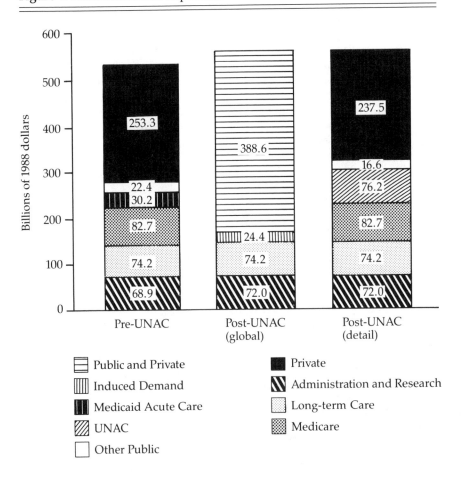

gram. If all employers chose to provide insurance rather than pay the X_1 fee, the number in the program could be as small as 42.9 million.[10]

The Technical Appendix I, *Financing Access To The Health Care System—Expenditures, Revenues, and Persons Covered*, presents detailed estimates of the coverage and benefits under UNAC as well as financing options. The following table provides a "snap-shot" of the plan estimates. For an in-depth analysis of the Commission's proposal, please see Technical Appendix I.

COST SHARING

Individual responsibility is a hallmark of the Commission's model health care system. By expanding access to 37 million Americans without health insurance, the Commission's model would enable the United States to join the rest of the developed world in assuring basic health care for its people. The Commission has offered a series of proposals for sharing the burden of health care costs in a way which assures access while encouraging rational economic choices.

The Commission is in favor of making consumers aware of the cost of their health care and is in favor of cost sharing for all Americans. But it recognizes that, for some Americans, cost sharing may create economic barriers that dissuade people from seeking needed health care. There-

Table 1: A Snap-Shot of Estimated Fees and Premiums[a] (in 1988 figures; estimates include administrative costs)

		Basic-option[b]	*Low-option[b]*
Pay only in absence of health insurance	X_1 fee (employer)	9.68%	8.75%
	X_2 fee (employee)	2.04%	1.85%
Everyone pays (includes health services research)	Y premium (employer)	0.68%	0.58%
	Y premium (employee)	0.66%	0.56%

[a]The X_1 fee is a percentage of wages and salaries up to $45,000. The X_2 fee and the Y premium are a percentage of adjusted gross income up to $45,000.
[b]These different benefit plans are described in Technical Appendix I.

---

[10]This is a very rough estimate, including: 6.9 of 37.4 million uninsured (the uninsured nonworkers who are not dependents of workers); 21 of 22.1 million Medicaid recipients; 2.7 of 19.5 million non-group insurance beneficiaries (who do not work); and 12.3 million uninsured part-year workers (who would be in the program part year and in an employer plan part year).

fore, the Commission has suggested a series of cost sharing mechanisms which will encourage rational economic behavior without denying necessary care.

In developing recommendations about the cost sharing provisions of the UNAC program, the Commission was particularly concerned that no provision be so burdensome that it denies access to necessary care. Equally important was a recognition that these beneficiaries will be a more economically diverse population than the current Medicaid population. Therefore, waiving some cost sharing provisions may make sense for low income participants but not necessarily for everyone in the program. However, the Commission was also guided by a desire for a system that was relatively simple to administer. The recommendations that follow are guidelines for the state agencies to utilize as they develop the programs within their states. The Commission encourages the private sector to follow suit.

The Commission's recommendations for the cost sharing provisions of the program were developed with full knowledge of the research on the effectiveness of cost sharing. Most of the evidence on the effect of cost sharing resulted from the major RAND Health Insurance Experiment (HIE). (5) The HIE results indicate that the use of medical services is influenced by the amount of money paid out-of-pocket. For example, the RAND studies showed that per capita expenses on a plan which required no out-of-pocket expenditures are 45 percent higher than those on a plan with a 95 percent coinsurance rate, subject to a $1,000 limit on out-of-pocket expenses. Cost sharing affects the number of medical contacts such as physician visits, but not the intensity of diagnostic tests or therapeutic services. Once a person is admitted, the use of hospital services is not affected by cost sharing.

The RAND study also indicated that the average person's health status changed very little, despite large increases in use associated with more generous coverage. Families with the most generous coverage spent about 50 percent more than families with the least generous coverage. There were some exceptions, however. Low-income, sick individuals did improve in health status. Free care was successful in reducing hypertension. In general, more encounters with physicians did not affect smoking, weight or cholesterol levels.

Cost Sharing Provisions: For the UNAC Program

Our cost sharing provisions were designed to control health care costs by making consumers more aware of them. The rest of this chapter describes how the three major cost sharing mechanisms—deductibles, copayments, and shared premiums—would be applied in the UNAC program.

1. Deductibles. Deductibles are designed to offset the payout of the first covered benefit. Most health insurance policies have relatively low deductibles, in the range of $50 to $200. (6) However, there is growing evidence that, in the future, deductibles in private insurance will increase to keep premiums affordable. The Commission therefore recommends that state agencies design their UNAC programs with a flexible deductible system, e.g., no deductible for low income groups and a higher deductible for those with higher income.

2. Coinsurance and Copayments. Both coinsurance and flat copayments are "point of service" (6) charges, or charges made at the time of service. Coinsurance refers to a fixed percentage of total charges for which the beneficiary or insured person is responsible. This is commonly set at 20 percent of the total medical bill, often paid after the insurance company pays the provider. The second type, the flat copayment, tends to be a small payment paid as services are rendered. These are most common in Health Maintenance Organizations and some medical plans, which may require a $2–5 fee for physician services or a $3 fee for a prescription drug.

Regarding coinsurance, the Commission recommends that the UNAC program design its coinsurance system more in line with the type of service provided rather than the site of care. This recognizes that under the current health care system, similar health services can be provided in a variety of settings and the old separation of reimbursement between inpatient and outpatient is no longer relevant. As a model, the Commission used a coinsurance rate of 20 percent for most services and a rate of 50 percent for outpatient mental health services, but this should only be viewed as a suggestion.

As an alternative, the Commission offers a recommendation for flat copayments. One approach is for state agencies to establish some copayment scheme. To assist poor people in meeting these payments, the Commission recommends that state agencies limit the amount of out-of-pocket costs based on per capita income. Such limits should both protect low income participants from high out-of-pocket costs and at the same time maintain incentives for cost consciousness. Setting out-of-pocket limits that vary with family income will be a complicated task requiring administrative control systems. But such limits are important if the Commission's Principle of Universal Access is to be followed.

Regardless of the cost-sharing method, the Commission recommends a limit on out-of-pocket expenses of $1,000 per person and $3,000 per family for the national package of basic services only. Any additional expenses would be the responsibility of the individual or the individual's employer insurance plan. These out-of-pocket limits could be cut in half for those under the poverty level.

The Commission also recommends that a method be devised to reduce or eliminate copayments for prenatal care, and perhaps other preventive services, in order to encourage wider use of preventive practices. It has been shown that for every one dollar invested in prenatal care, over three dollars are saved. (7)

3. Shared Premiums. Consistent with the Commission's Principles of Shared Responsibility and Universal Access, UNAC beneficiaries above 150 percent of the poverty level would share in the premium by paying the X_2 fee, while those below would not pay a fee.

Cost Sharing Provisions: For the Private Sector

The Commission supports the increased cost sharing that has developed in the private sector over the last few years and encourages additional progress in this regard. The Commission urges cost-sharing innovations designed to establish economic constraints that encourage rational decisionmaking without compromising access to health care.

In recent years, for example, employees have paid a greater share of health insurance premiums. (8) Shared premiums are more common for policies which cover families than for individual policies, because premiums for individual policies rarely exceed the caps that employers set on the amount of premium they will pay for each employee. Employees are required to contribute to only 25 percent of conventional health insurance plans for individual policies, while they have to contribute to almost half of conventional insurance plans covering families. (8)

Recent data indicate that employees are willing to pay a portion of higher HMO or PPO premiums in comparison to conventional insurance premiums, in exchange for lower point-of-service payments. (8) Employees with conventional insurance pay about 25 percent of the family plan premium; those with an HMO family plan pay on average 26 percent of the premium, and those covered by a PPO family plan 31 percent of the premium. (9)

In an effort to achieve cost sensitivity, some large employers have increased their deductibles to the $1,000 to $3,000 range, which suggests that their insurance plans could be characterized as catastrophic coverage. (7)(9)(10) In order to promote preventive care and appropriate early intervention, the Commission suggests that cost sharing in the private

Table 2: Recommended Cost-Sharing Provisions for the UNAC Program[1] and the Private Sector

	Premium	Deductibles	Coinsurance[2] and co-payment			Out-of-Pocket Limits
			Covered charges for in-patient hospital and mental health care	Inpatient and outpatient physician care	Outpatient mental health care	
Employer-provided coverage	Employee pays no more than 25% of premium –or– Employer is subject to X_1 fee	Left to the determination of the marketplace				
UNAC program beneficiaries above 150% of the federal poverty level	The X_2 fee is the employee's share of the premium (i.e., ensures the individual of UNAC program coverage)	Small deductible	A small percent	20% up to the negotiated amount	50% up to the negotiated amount	$1,000 per person, $3,000 per family for the National Package of Basic Services
UNAC program beneficiaries at or below 150% of the federal poverty level	Subsidized by the program	Small deductible	Adjusted according to ability to pay; must pay something	Adjusted according to ability to pay; must pay something	$500 per person	$1,500 per family for National Package of Basic Services

[1]These are only recommendations; the ultimate decision rests with the state agencies.
[2]Alternatively, this could be flat co-payments.

sector should parallel cost-sharing provisions in the UNAC program, i.e., vary by income, for low-income employees.

Establishing and Updating the National Package of Basic Benefits

The process of establishing a national basic benefits package would generate significant debate. Hearings or public testimony could be akin to a "town hall" debate on important medical, ethical, and legal issues related to difficult choices ranging from neonatal intensive care to heroic therapeutic treatments for the very old. It is important to have an ongoing, national forum in which to deliberate these issues; one of the few certainties in health policy is that we, as a nation, will always face these choices.

The initial package of basic benefits should be set by enabling legislation. The Commission strongly recommends that mental health benefits and preventive services, especially prenatal care, be included in this package.

The role of the National Quality Improvement Initiative would be to recommend biennially to Congress how best to update the basic benefits in the national package. It is essential that it be done on a permanent, ongoing basis. The Commission recommends including this function in the National Quality Improvement Initiative in order to facilitate access to the most recent information on quality and costs.

Once the national benefits package is determined, employers and individuals purchasing their own insurance would, of course, be free to supplement it. In addition, states could require that the basic level of benefits be higher for their residents, for both private and program beneficiaries.

Funding of Health Services Research

The Commission's plan includes funding research to develop guidelines for health services. This research would be funded with a supplemental fee applied to the Y premium for both employers and individuals. We estimate that to fund $500 million in research per year, the rate applied to both the employer and the employee Y revenue bases would be about one-tenth of one percent (0.11 percent). (11) This amount is included in the estimates presented earlier in the chapter.

While the Commission agreed that an earmarked portion of the Y premium was the best approach for funding additional health services research, a number of other approaches were considered. The Commissioners recognized that a recommendation for an additional payment would be extremely difficult, given the current political climate. At the same time, however, there was no area that achieved greater consensus than the need to learn more about ways to improve and to document the value of our care. It was widely agreed, too, that an insufficient amount of resources, both dollars and people, have gone into this effort. Even these resources have led to startling and disturbing discoveries about the amount of inappropriate care being delivered in the case of several expensive procedures.

A number of Commissioners discussed the merits of using funds from general revenues. However, to signify best the importance of health services research, and to provide assurance that the funds will indeed be available for this work (given the competition for today's limited dollars), the Commissioners felt that the earmarked Y premium was an equitable approach. The fact that the amount of the premium in question would be so small—about one-tenth of one percent (0.11 percent)—lends further support to the Commissioners' recommendation.

Another funding alternative considered but rejected by the majority of Commissioners because of its regressive nature was some type of user fee channeled through the U.S. Treasury. Because all care would have, at least theoretically, the benefit of the information generated, the user fee could be a surcharge on all claims filed, public and private. The main disadvantage with this approach is that only the sick (users of care) instead of all individuals (the potentially sick) would fund the research that would benefit everyone at some point in life.

REFERENCES

1. Porkony, J., "Report on Health Care," *Health Management Quarterly* 10(1):5, 1988.
2. Callahan, D., "Allocating Health Resources," *Center Report*, April/May 1988, p. 18.
3. Etheredge, L., Reinhardt, U., et al., "Hard Choices in Health Care: A Matter of Ethics," *Health Care: How to Improve It and Pay For It*, Center for National Policy, Washington, DC, April 1985.
4. Enthoven, A., in his paper, *A Consumer Choice Health Plan for the 1990s: A Proposal for Universal Health Insurance*, February 3, 1988.
5. Manning, W., Newhouse, J., et al., *Health Insurance and the Demand for Medical Care: Evidence from a Randomized Experiment*, RAND Research Report, R 3476-HHS, February 1988.
6. Rosou, J., and Zayer, R., *Improving Health Care Management in the Workplace*, Pergamon Press, 1985.
7. Institute of Medicine, *Preventing Low Birthweight*, National Academy Press, Washington, DC, 1985.

8. Prospective Payment Assessment Commission, *Medicare Prospective Payment and the American Health Care System: Report to the Congress*, U.S. Government Printing Office, Washington, DC, June 1988, p. 99.

9. Hewitt Associates, "Salaried Employee Benefits Provided by Major U.S. Employers in 1986," *Medical Benefits*, June 15, 1987.

10. Shapiro, M., personal communication to Campbell, P., The Lash Group.

11. Lewin/ICF, Inc., *Expenditures and Revenues Under an Illustrative Universal Health Coverage Plan*, prepared for the National Leadership Commission on Health Care, September 27, 1988.

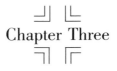

Chapter Three

Cost Control and Quality Improvement: State and Local Initiatives

Interrelated problems, especially in our complex health care system, cry out for interrelated solutions. And such solutions naturally need a systemic strategy to succeed. Such a strategy in a health care system as diverse and in need of reform as ours is not easy to design or implement.

The challenge in building such a strategy is to blend the strengths of local innovation with leadership and coordination from the state and national levels. A first step is to assign responsibilities for all parties—providers and patients, employers and employees, payers and insurers, the private and public sectors, physicians and other health professionals, and federal and state governments. The next step is to create mechanisms that encourage all parties to carry out their responsibilities.

In early discussions about cost control methods designed to impose economic discipline on the health care system,[1] the Commission looked carefully at past cost containment policies. (1) Accepting Stuart Altman's characterization that the present system is in "the twilight zone between competition and regulation," (2) the Commission concluded that it was both philosophically sound and realistic to adopt an approach blending competitive and regulatory strategies. A prominent precedent is Medicare's Prospective Payment System (PPS), affecting about 40 per-

---

[1]Lawrence Lewin has defined the cost containment problem as "the challenge of imposing economic discipline on health care markets. By way of definition, an economically disciplined market is one in which neither providers nor consumers of health care services are allowed to pass the cost of their mistakes or abusive behavior onto others with impunity." (1)

cent of all hospital business; it pays hospitals a pre-determined amount for each person's hospital stay based on the person's diagnosis. PPS can be viewed as regulatory, when the focus is on governmentally-set prices, or as competitive, when the focus is on hospital incentives for efficiency, or on the impact of a powerful prudent purchaser. PPS's dual approach has clearly succeeded in stemming the rate of growth of hospital expenditures.[2]

Weighing the generally mixed results of competition and regulation in terms of controlling costs, ensuring access, and maintaining quality care, and mindful of the old adage that "where you stand depends on where you sit," the Commissioners reached a consensus in recommending a strategy that fosters the competitive efforts already begun in the public and private sectors, strengthens them with solid information, and establishes necessary controls to meet social goals and common interests.

After agreeing that there should be a national package of basic health care benefits to which every American has access, the Commissioners proposed allowing the states to determine any additional benefits for their residents. For the Universal Access program,[3] the Commission endorses a state entity administering the program, complete with the power to negotiate with providers and practitioners to establish the package and payment policies for the program beneficiaries.[4] The Commission explicitly chose where possible to work with existing state agencies rather than create a new level of bureaucracy.

Clearly the behavior of all parties (patients, payers, and providers) needs changing, and information about the effectiveness, outcomes, and costs of care needs to be far more available than in the past. In pursuit of this goal, the Commission discussed extensively the concept of an integrating mechanism on the state level with the legal authority to contract with the various payers (Federal government, state and local government, and business) to obtain for their beneficiaries the best possible care.

One mechanism the Commission recommends is leadership by a state agency in serving the collective interests of providers, practitioners, payers, and patients. The states have long acted as conduits between local and national concerns, and the Commission is comfortable with the concept of modifying a national priority to accommodate our heterogeneous population at the state level. Given variations among local pop-

---

[2]PPS has also had the effect of shifting more care to outpatient settings, which has contributed to an unprecedented rise in ambulatory expenditures. It is widely accepted that the result has been cost shifting. New policies must focus on all care, not just hospital care, if total costs are to be controlled.

[3]This model program, called the UNAC program, is a plan to finance access to a basic level of care for all Americans. It is described in depth in Chapter 2.

ulations within states, some states may want to vary their plans within their boundaries to allow for regional diversity. Our history is replete with examples of state-level experimentation that encourages flexibility and innovation.

The Commission recognizes the potential impact of the state's negotiating power on the private financing and delivery system, including the potential impact of information developed on quality or costs at the state level. By integrating and disseminating information needed by all parties, state agencies could play an important role in the interrelated goals of quality improvement and cost control, both national concerns with enough local and state differences to merit give and take between parties at all levels.

The Commission recommends that the designated agencies within the states provide leadership for all payers who wish to participate, public and private. As they administer a program that guarantees access to a national basic package of services, state agencies should provide leadership in accommodating the particular needs of their state residents; in serving as a prudent purchaser of health care, balancing cost and quality concerns; and in facilitating negotiation among different interests, guarding against excessive cost-shifting.

The Commission then deliberated about whether the state authority to administer UNAC and, in the process, to negotiate with providers and practitioners to set payment policies on behalf of UNAC beneficiaries, should be expanded to apply to the beneficiaries of all payers, including private business. Several Commissioners supported such expansion of the state role, asserting that such an all-payer system could be crucial to avert harmful cost-shifting. But in an effort to minimize mandating, the majority supported a more limited role, emphasizing that the role and composition of the state agency should be designed in such a way as to reduce cost-shifting concerns. Upon further reflection, some Commissioners expressed concern about the prospects of success for a proposal that would exclude private payers from the public negotiations. So a majority opted to recommend a compromise position that allows private payers to join at the outset of the new plan or a new rate-setting year and then be bound by the state agency's payment rate decisions and arrangements for provision of care.

THE STATE AGENCIES

The Commission recommends that states broaden a state agency to include representatives of the major private stakeholders in health care—

---

[4]The Commission also discussed at great length whether to allow a state agency to negotiate on behalf of all payers.

payers, providers, practitioners, and consumers—perhaps appointed by state governors. The Commission recognizes that it will not be easy to generate the cooperation needed to realize its goals, primarily because attitudes will have to change. A recent assessment by the Institute of Medicine of public health programs, which at least have a tradition requiring cooperation, lends support to this concern:

> Today, while numerous examples can be found of medical community support for public health activities, . . . too often, confrontation and suspicion are evident on both sides. For example, the director of one state medical association characterized the health department as distrustful of physicians, and cited the director's effort to push a mandatory data reporting system through the legislature without consulting the society. (3)

But the Commission is unanimously convinced that cooperation is both desirable and possible. It is clear to the Commission from its discussions with dozens of physicians and the testimony of leaders of the professions that they are eager to play a role in this process. The Commission regards their role as essential to the success of any proposed change in health care policy.

State administration of the UNAC program, including negotiating payment policies, should cost less than the cost of administering the current Medicaid program because the state agency would not have to determine eligibility.[5] The Commission recognizes that expanding representation in an agency would incur some additional costs.

To cover services for UNAC beneficiaries, states would receive funds on a per beneficiary basis from current Medicaid acute care funds, the X_1 and X_2 fees, and most of the Y premium payments. The amount could be estimated prospectively and reconciled at year's end. Current funds for administering the acute care portion of the Medicaid program would remain at these agencies. The calculation of the amounts needed to cover program beneficiaries includes the cost of administration.

The Commission recommends that the agencies rely whenever possible on contracts with private groups having experience in the various functional areas. One possible contract for a major function would be claims processing for program beneficiaries, which could be done by any third-party payer with that experience, such as insurance companies.

A state agency provides a structural connection between national

---

[5]Lewin/ICF estimates that the "pure" administrative costs for the pool will be about 8 percent. Insurance for small groups, however, often contains an administrative surcharge of 12 to 25 percent to account for the risk of a high-cost illness costing more than the premiums collected.

concerns and local preferences in the Commission's proposal, as well as one of the connections between the public and private sectors. The Commission intends the state agency to go beyond the role of a traditional agency and set examples in using the investment in information to enhance the competitive forces underway today. The state agency would not only administer the UNAC program, but as one of the largest payers in any state, it should also take a leadership role in both public and private payment policies, finding innovative uses for information developed about the outcomes, costs, and quality of care.

State agency negotiations with providers and practitioners to establish payment policies are likely to focus specifically on: the method by which hospitals and physicians are paid, how much they are paid, whether and by what criteria specific providers and practitioners are selected as preferred for preferential payment, and which utilization management policies will be part of the payment scheme. An agency should be encouraged to coordinate with Medicare payment policies whenever possible.

The Commissioners have repeatedly stressed the importance of negotiating *fair* rates for the strategy to work. If paying for care for all Americans becomes explicit on the financing side of the health care equation, it is necessary to do away with extensive cost shifting on the delivery side. This could be accomplished in mandatory or voluntary ways. The majority of Commissioners opted to recommend, at least initially, a voluntary approach with all policies and rates negotiated by the state to be in the public domain. Thus, all payers will have the opportunity to use this information in their own negotiations, or alternatively, to volunteer in advance to be bound by the states' decisions.

Many state agencies are likely to place physician payment reform high on their agendas. Early in its deliberations, the Commission reached consensus on the need to modify physician payment, including paying physicians more for time spent with patients, and providing financial incentives for physicians (and hospitals) to use information on appropriateness and quality. Certainly, the Commission urges a careful examination of the use of the relative value scale developed by William Hsiao and colleagues and currently under review by the Physician Payment Review Commission (PPRC) and HCFA. The Commission hopes state agencies will build on this work and take a leadership role in its application.

Armed with information from the National Quality Improvement Initiative—including guidelines about the appropriateness of medical practices and, before too long, information about what makes a high quality provider—the Commission expects the state agency to act as prudent purchasers of care, in part by selecting providers for program beneficiaries. State agencies can encourage the use of multiple utilization management techniques, including preadmission screening, concurrent review, and second surgical opinions. There is new evidence that these techniques can indeed help to manage costs. In order to assure quality, they could be based, where appropriate, on the new practice guidelines that will be developed.

The state agency may also want to consider contracting with pre-ferred provider organizations (PPOs) and health maintenance organizations (HMOs). In 1987, in the private sector, 32 percent of Americans with private group insurance were in managed fee-for-service plans, 16 percent were in an HMO, and 11 percent were in a PPO, leaving only 41 percent in unmanaged fee-for-service. (4)

These methods, combined with the payment policy and rate negotiations, are important but go only so far toward controlling costs. For example, HMOs achieve cost reductions through the use of fewer hospital days, PPOs receive discounts from hospitals, and managed fee-for-service uses prospective utilization review. The weakness is that these methods focus solely on inpatient care. We still need to develop ways to control the cost of ever-increasing outpatient services.

An interesting idea—the use of "expenditure targets"—is gaining support among policy makers concerned with rising costs and is worth exploring further.[6] The idea is to set a target budget that would be allowed to rise for inflation and growth in beneficiaries, but if the year's rate of usage exceeds the target, then there would be a lower adjustment in rates in the following year. For the UNAC program, the negotiation of physician fees lends itself particularly well to expenditure targets. Although the concept is not fully developed, it has a certain appeal, as noted recently by Dr. Philip Caper of Dartmouth College: "Once a cost limit has been set, politicians, purchasers of private health insurance, and consultants would no longer be involved in determining what is best for an individual patient. That decision would be sent back where it belongs—to the doctor and patient." (5)

The state agency should conduct an ongoing evaluation of its programs, in keeping with the theme of continual improvement. Information developed about what works and what does not should be used to modify that state's program. Each evaluation should examine the impact of payment policies on key players in the system, for both UNAC and private payer beneficiaries. The agency may wish to monitor any impacts of the program on physician supply and on charges to private beneficiaries.

---

[6]This idea was developed in PPRC's March 1988 report to the Congress.

ADDITIONAL STATE AND LOCAL ACTIVITIES

There are important developments in the area of the quality of care that public and private organizations at the state and local levels should be aware of. Brook and Kosecoff (6) proposed the following principles of a quality assessment system that the Commission has found useful: We need to tolerate public acknowledgement of differences in quality among health care systems; quality assessment of a system is a public good. Such quality assessments should emphasize populations of patients and physicians rather than focus on individuals.

And quality assessments should be conducted for the purpose of improvement, not punishment. As noted recently by Commission Adviser Dennis O'Leary, President of the Joint Commission on Accreditation of Healthcare Organizations (JCAHO), ". . .[Q]uality assessment is a vehicle for reaching loftier yet fundamental objectives, the elimination or reduction in aberrances of care, and the improved provision of care that is already reasonably well performed. These objectives can be attained only through the appropriate gathering and use of information that has been determined through physician expertise to be relevant to clinical performance and the quality of care." (7)

Although assessments should focus on improvement, they can reveal serious problems. Witness the findings of a new RAND Corporation study that as many as one-quarter of the deaths of patients with heart ailments, stroke and pneumonia in 12 hospitals could have been prevented—the study found that physicians made a variety of errors in the diagnosis and treatment of such patients. (8) Such studies only highlight the need to develop more and better information for public use.

Medicare's Peer Review Organizations (PROs) can and should expand their quality measurement efforts. For example, the Illinois Peer Review Organization is going to use certain standards of medical practice in cases of possible myocardial infarction patients and when antibiotics are prescribed. This new program was based on their research that found wide variation in medical practice patterns for monitoring patients with chest pain. First, the PRO will establish guidelines for these areas. Then it plans to develop and conduct continuing education programs for physicians and nurses. This represents a sharp departure for some PROs: in the past, most PRO efforts have been directed at isolating cases of poor quality and taking action, rather than at educating. (9)

Other current efforts abound that will produce benefits at the state and local levels: the JCAHO serves to measure some aspects of quality. Manufacturers have responded to hospital interest in economic information on their products and the cost-effective use of those products. The American Medical Review Research Center and Codman Research

Group have a project on developing ways PROs can communicate small-area analysis to practicing physicians. Numerous medical societies have quality assessment and improvement projects. Physicians have responded to the new information and, indeed, in most cases are the ones that have developed it.

The Commission urges the state agency to be aware of programs for widespread education led by state medical societies about appropriateness and quality guidelines developed under the new quality initiative. This information should include clear statements of both guideline policies and the rationales for them, including the evidence, outcomes, and reasoning. The Commission believes that even with increased and improved utilization management, any attempts to control the volume of services will depend on the attitude of the general public towards foregoing medical procedures of uncertain value. Public education over time is once again the key.

Once guidelines have been accepted as credible, hospitals and individual physicians still need to decide how they should be adapted to a particular area. After years of studying the use of medical information by practicing physicians, Ann Greer has found it intrinsically difficult for knowledge emanating from external sources to affect local behavior. Only local innovators and committed idea champions can really reach local opinion leaders and their constituencies, irrespective of the esteem accorded the new knowledge. (10) The role of state medical societies and medical journals in this effort will be crucial.

Local managed care systems could encourage innovative ways of applying industrial quality control techniques to health care. (11) They could sponsor a project that "translates" industrial quality control terms to language understood by health care providers. They could establish a prize for those health care organizations most committed to quality improvement, similar to the National Baldridge Prize for quality in American business. Indicators for selection would include: the commitment of the organization's CEO and trustees to improving quality, the use of modern statistical methods to set priorities for problem solving, a minimal amount of "waste, rework, and complexity," and an atmosphere where the punishment factor is removed from collected data on quality outcomes, among others.

Establishing State-Wide Supplemental Benefits

As noted throughout this report, the Commission felt strongly that every American should be ensured access to a basic package of services established nationally. With the clear intention that the package should represent necessary and not "Cadillac" care, the Commission recommends that it be designed to be as comprehensive as possible and to include preventive care, especially prenatal services, and mental health care. By definition, that package is considered a floor in health care beneath which no American will be permitted to sink. As noted in Chapter 2, the primary rationale for folding Medicaid into the Commission's program is the great variation in benefits and eligibility that exists among state Medicaid programs.

The Commission discussed at length whether the states should be permitted to supplement the national basic package, and if so, whether those additional benefits would apply to the program only or would also be considered in determining whether an employer's package met the minimum. The majority felt that the traditional state privilege of supplementing a Federal program should remain, and therefore the states should be empowered to establish state-wide supplemental benefits.

IMPLICATIONS FOR COST CONTROL

The Commission's cost control strategy has an excellent chance of succeeding if adopted across the board, much less chance if implemented in a piecemeal fashion. First, the Commission calls for allowing the competitive advances of the past few years to play out further, with the addition of a greater investment in usable information that is called for under the National Quality Improvement Initiative. It allows for flexibility on a local basis to meet needs of the consumers, payers, providers, and practitioners in the area. In essence, a restructuring of the marketplace could occur.

State agencies, as large payers, can be an important force for cost control in several ways, including: their ability to negotiate payment policies for the new program (and other payers who join voluntarily); their ability to select providers as a "prudent purchaser"; and their leadership in serving as models for using national practice guidelines to improve the value of care (e.g., in precertification programs) or for creating model payment policies or expenditure targets.

These are powerful tools that could have a significant impact on the private sector. Payers' and providers' representation in the state agencies should further encourage fair cost control. Any selective contracting that blends cost and quality concerns should be done with an explicit under-' standing of cross-over effects to the private sector.

There are many other lessons, of course, but perhaps the most important one is that cost control measures taken by any group acting alone are unlikely to have an impact on national expenditures, although they might well affect that group. Furthermore, any effective measures will be painful for some and difficult for many in the absence of strong involvement of state and local providers.

Evidence from our Canadian neighbors tells us that fee controls that are not backed up by some form of global payment caps can be only partially successful in controlling costs, especially when coupled with an increasing supply of physicians. But even if fee levels, utilization, and supply are all addressed, policies must reflect "some degree of administrative intelligence, backed up with political will and applied through an ongoing negotiation process," if they are to work. (12)

REFERENCES

1. Lewin, L., *Cost Containment Until Today: Lessons for Tomorrow,* paper prepared for the National Leadership Commission on Health Care, May 1988, p. 1.
2. Altman, S., "The American Healthcare System: The Twilight Zone Between Competition and Regulation," *Emerging Issues in Health Care,* Estes Park Institute, Englewood, CA, 1988, pp. 7–11.
3. Institute of Medicine, *The Future of Public Health: Summary and Recommendations,* p. xvii, August 1988, prepublication copy.
4. Gabel, J., Jajich-Toth, C., et al., "The Changing World of Group Health Insurance," *Health Affairs* 7(3):48–65, Summer 1988, p. 54.
5. Caper, P., "Solving the Medical Care Dilemma," *NEJM* 318(23):1535–1536, June 9, 1988, p. 1536.
6. Brook, R., and Kosecoff, J., "Competition and Quality," *Health Affairs* 7(3):150–161, Summer 1988.
7. O'Leary, D., "Quality Assessment: Moving from Theory to Practice," *JAMA* 260(12):1760, September 23/30, 1988.
8. "News at Deadline," *Hospitals,* 62(20):12, October 20, 1988 (reporting on a study reported in the October 3, 1988 edition of *Annals of Internal Medicine*).
9. "PRO's Use Medical Practice Standards to Assess Quality," *Hospitals* 62(20):19–20, October 20, 1988.
10. Greer, A., "The State of the Art Versus the State of the Science: The Diffusion of New Medical Technologies into Practice," *International Journal of Technology Assessment in Health Care* 4(1):5–26, 1988.
11. Berwick, D., *Measuring Health Care Quality,* unpublished paper MS# PR40-87/88, Harvard Community Health Plan, September 21, 1987, p. 19.
12. Barer, M., Evans, R., and Labelle, R., "Fee Controls as Cost Control: Tales from the Frozen North," *Milbank Quarterly* 66(1):1–64, 1988.

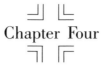

Chapter Four

A National Quality Improvement Initiative: A New Unifying Strategy

What is quality health care? One definition the Commission found useful describes it as:

> the performance of specific activities in a manner that either decreases or at least prevents the deterioration in health status that would have occurred as a function of a disease or condition. Employing this definition, quality of care consists of two components: 1) the selection of the right activity or task or combination of activities, and 2) the performance of those activities in manner that produces the best outcome. (1)

Quality goes beyond technical care to include the interpersonal interaction between the patient and those providing care; continuity of care among different providers is also an important factor. Quality care requires integrating the skills of practitioners with the capabilities of health care organizations (such as hospitals, nursing homes, and managed care plans) and with wise local, state, and national health care policies. Clearly, the concepts of quality (in its more narrow sense), appropriateness, and effectiveness are intertwined. When referring to care provided, the Commission often uses quality in its broadest sense to encompass all these concepts.

The Commission's work has occurred at the same time that concerted attention is being given by leading organizations to understanding and addressing the problems in the quality and appropriateness of health care services. Experts at the forefront of this rapidly expanding body of work provided the Commission with information on the latest developments in such critical areas as health care quality measures, appropriateness of health care services, practice pattern variation, outcomes research, the application of industrial quality control techniques to health care, and the use of large-scale data bases to characterize and stimulate improvement in the science and practice of medicine.

THE NEED FOR A QUALITY IMPROVEMENT INITIATIVE

Many theories and programs exist for improving quality and appropriateness, and many work well. Many researchers and increasing numbers of health care providers, payers, and patients are involved in these activities. What has led the Commission to propose a new unifying strategy for a national quality improvement initiative?

The Commission has concluded that an important level of inappropriate over- and under use of care has been documented for some time now. The reasons for inappropriate care include the following: an incomplete and continually evolving science base for that care, often creating uncertainty about appropriateness and effectiveness in clinical decisionmaking; perverse financial incentives; seeking to meet unrealistically high patient expectations; and the malpractice crisis. In addition, systems for assuring that care is provided in the best possible fashion are too often inadequate.

Health professionals and patients need several types of new knowledge. When a consensus on medical knowledge is possible, they need to learn better which tests and procedures are appropriate for an individual situation. When guidelines exist for particular conditions or treatments, they need to understand the scientific basis of those guidelines. They also need more basic scientific information about which medical practices are truly effective and which are not. And they need better ways to measure what happens when care is provided and how it can be more effective.

Improving information on quality and appropriateness will have far-reaching effects. In addition to reducing the level of uncertainty, which, in turn, reduces unnecessary and inappropriate care, improvements in quality and appropriateness information should also help stem the tide of increasing health care costs, increase efficiency, improve the doctor-patient relationship, and reduce malpractice suits.

Fortunately, there is solid evidence that health care providers will use relevant, well-presented information to improve the quality and appropriateness of their care. The Commission has discovered that governmental agencies and private organizations with clinical expertise are actively pursuing:

1. Objective cataloging of the proper use of existing and emerging approaches to diagnosis and treatment, often known as appropriateness research and technology assessment;

2. Clinical trials on the effectiveness of medical practices;

3. Research designed to understand and, where appropriate, reduce practice variation, often known as outcomes research and practice pattern monitoring;

4. Synthesis of current research and clinical experience into useful practice guidelines; and

5. Development and use of clinical and organizational measures to stimulate improvement in the quality and appropriateness of care.

Examples of these activities can be found in Appendix C. Together they represent an essential and unprecedented commitment to improving health care. There is no lack of innovation and useful alternative perspectives.

What the Commission has found, however, is woeful underfunding of every component of the work identified above and ineffective coordination. The Commission found lacking a process where participants can step outside their own organization's interest to help develop a nationally coordinated strategy. The Commissioners have agreed that such a strategy would ideally involve periodic collective priority setting, coordination, and progress evaluation, while maintaining decentralized activities.

The need for coordination is evident in the fact, for example, that over 65 organizations are working in the area of technology assessment alone, according to the Institute of Medicine's (IOM) Council on Health Care Technology. (2) While the Commission expects the IOM's role to continue and be expanded, it feels that there is a distinct relationship between technology assessment and other activities—such as developing guidelines about appropriateness and quality, and synthesizing information on clinical and health outcomes—and that the relationship is sufficient to warrant additional coordination and facilitation. Recent Federal activities in the areas of appropriateness and effectiveness are divided among several agencies, with the Health Care Financing Administration (HCFA) and the National Center for Health Services Research and Health Care Technology Assessment (NCHSR) *both* having leading roles, carried out very differently.

ACTION—A NEW, UNIFYING QUALITY IMPROVEMENT INITIATIVE

The Commission strongly recommends a major new National Quality Improvement Initiative—that will expand and unify currently uncoordinated work in developing and disseminating information about effectiveness, appropriateness, quality, and costs of care.

Dr. Edmund Pellegrino, one of the Commissioners, once said that "[M]edicine is the most humane of the arts, the most artistic of the sciences, and the most scientific of the humanities." (3) How can this artistic science become a more scientific art? There are a number of ways. The Commission proposes four key goals for this initiative:

1. A major expansion of information about the quality (efficacy, appropriateness, effectiveness, technical performance and continuity) of health care services;
2. Development and continual enhancement of national practice guidelines for appropriate medical practices, useful to practitioners and patients in making decisions;
3. Significant growth in the development of rigorous measures of health care quality and practice guides for using these measures in day-to-day quality improvement;
4. Widespread dissemination of the above information.

The Commission believes that these objectives together form the framework for a new or renewed culture which will foster continuous improvement in our health care system. The health care industry is beginning to look toward other industries for lessons in quality. Successful industries have, in many cases, learned that high quality depends on continual improvement. They find that quality measurement is best guided by a firm conviction that one can be better tomorrow than today. An institution should not attempt to prove that it is good enough now and need not improve. Quality control should be grounded in aspiration, not in defense. (4) The Commission believes that these ideas apply to the entire quality area as we have defined it, including appropriateness, efficiency, and more traditional "quality" concepts.

Achieving these objectives will take not only time, but also sufficient and predictable funding, wise priority setting and progress evaluation, integration of public and private efforts, and demonstrable openness and objectivity. These ingredients for success are discussed briefly below.

Sufficient and Predictable Funding

This National Quality Improvement Initiative is a major effort justified by this nation's substantial investment in health care and by the importance of good health to the fulfillment of both individual and national potential.

The Commission is calling for an annual increase of investment rising gradually to about $500 million per year to be obtained from an earmarked portion of the Y premium described in Chapter 2.[1] The $500 million figure is in addition to funding which must continue to be provided for clinical research, including randomized clinical trials. As currently estimated, the Y health premium rate paid by all American individuals above 150 percent of the Federal poverty level and all employers, private and governmental, would increase by .11 to fund this investment. This approach is another example of the Commission's philosophy that we as citizens have a "shared responsibility" to provide high quality health care, to all Americans.

At the Commission's request, Lewin/ICF prepared a very rough estimate of potential savings that could be generated by reducing inappropriate care.[2] Based on HCFA estimates that as much as two percentage points of the annual hospital intensity index would be influenced by practice pattern changes, the Commission's estimate suggests a potential saving of two percentage points of the currently projected growth rate of health expenditure. This means that over a four-year period, about $5.9 billion annually for Medicare Parts A and B combined could be influenced by changes in practice pattern. For national health expenditures, the figure is $84 billion for fiscal years 1990–1993, or an average of $22 billion annually that could be influenced by practice pattern changes. Using a second method of approximating the potential effects of changing practice patterns on health care costs, the Commission developed a very conservative "bottom up" estimate of potential savings from reducing inappropriate services; assuming a 4 percent growth rate in health expenditures annually, this estimate could approach $1.5 billion a year by FY 93.

Earmarking a portion of the Y premium as the funding mechanism for health services research would provide a stable, permanent source of funding for this important work. The underlying principle of this ap-

---

[1] For comparison purposes, the amount spent by HCFA and NCHSR together in FY 1988 in this field was $47 million. These agencies provide the bulk of funding along with some private foundation monies.

[2] See Technical Appendix III for complete estimate.

proach is that information on the effectiveness, outcome, and cost-effectiveness, as well as recommended guidelines on when to use a test should be an easily accessible public good. Since everyone supports improving health care, information on how to do so is clearly a public good, both in the everyday sense and in the specialized sense used by economists. (5) Because such information is widely perceived as a social good, the cost and the benefits of it should be widely shared.

The Commission considered predictability for this funding critically important. Past and current underfunding of this work will discourage the small body of currently trained researchers and cause educational institutions to avoid developing the graduate level programs necessary to train the large cadre of individuals needed to pursue these objectives for the next several decades.

As noted below, funding should flow through those organizations and agencies that have demonstrated their capability and which meet criteria for objectivity, openness and fiscal responsibility.

Wise Priority Setting and Progress Evaluation

The magnitude of this National Quality Improvement Initiative demands wise and continual priority setting. While it could be argued that high priority needs are easily identified—based, for example, on criteria such as risk to patients, dollars spent, and perceived quality problems—it would be prudent to establish priorities in a deliberate fashion. Only then can the returns on our investment in information eventually be measured.

The Commission recommends that a process be established to identify priority activities for each of the four objectives noted above. This process should occur annually or every two years. It should be guided by the types of criteria noted in the preceding paragraph. And it should involve knowledgeable individuals who provide care, direct quality improvement programs, and conduct related research, as well as those who receive, insure and purchase care. High priority activities should represent a mix of short-term and long-term projects.

Similarly, this process should periodically look at progress made in realizing the objectives. This function would also serve to analyze levels of funding for research in the public and private sectors and make judgments as to their adequacy.

Integrating Public and Private Skills and Responsibilities

The Commission considered several options for organizing and overseeing the extensive activities needed to improve the quality and appropriateness of health care. These options ranged from creating a new national oversight and coordinating body to channeling more funds to current organizations, without changing their configuration, processes, or interactions.

The Commission rejected both of these options. Rather, it recommends building on current expertise, giving much more attention to the methodologic rigor, objectivity, and openness of existing research; development, dissemination and implementation projects; and more focus on coordination among them. By expanding and improving what exists, we can more rapidly attack our problems and avoid creating a duplicative and expensive bureaucracy.

As noted earlier, the success of this National Quality Improvement Initiative is dependent on adequate, long-term funding, wise priority setting and progress evaluation, objective research and development (across the spectrum of activities described above), rapid dissemination of research results, development of practice guidelines based on the research, and timely integration of new knowledge into day-to-day practice. The following table illustrates some of the organizations that have demonstrated their capability in each of these areas.[3] Coordination would occur through the priority setting process, which would be facilitated by an organization, such as the IOM, with expertise in this area.

Table 1: Examples of Organizations Involved in Quality Improvement

Activity	*Agency/Organization*
Funding	Dept. of Health and Human Services (NIH, NCHSR, HCFA)
Priority setting	Institute of Medicine
R&D	Universities Private research organizations American Medical Association (AMA) JCAHO HCFA; PHS (NCHSR, HRSA, NIH)
Information dissemination	Medical journals AMA PHS (NCHSR, HRSA) Medical specialty associations
Guidelines development	AMA Medical specialty associations
Stimulating integration into practice	JCAHO Medical societies

---

[3]These organizations are listed as examples of organizations with particular capabilities. The Commission does not intend to imply that they are the only organizations with those capabilities or that each organization can perform only the functions listed.

This table makes it clear that health care leaders are committed to understanding and improving the quality of care and that their organizations have the expertise to meet this challenge. What we lack is adequate funding and a process which ensures that the infusion of resources is coordinated and used wisely, and that the results from all these diverse organizations are made widely available throughout the professions, not just in those specialities for which they are primarily intended.

The Commission believes that effective investment can be assured through the following measures:

1. Creation of an expanded fund secured under a shared responsibility from health insurance premiums (a small portion of the Commission's proposed Y health premium).

2. Legislative sanction for a public-private partnership, such as the Institute of Medicine, to bring together periodically knowledgeable individuals who provide care, direct quality improvement programs, and conduct related research, as well as those who receive, insure and purchase care, the purpose being to identify the highest priority research and development activities for each of the four objectives noted earlier. This process would also be charged with periodically evaluating progress of this Initiative. It could be assisted by the creation of a finite-term blue-ribbon advisory group, similar in stature to the Health Insurance Benefits Advisory Committee established in 1965 when Medicare and Medicaid were born, to examine the progress of this initiative and report periodically to the President, Congress, and the American People.

3. Legislative requirements that the targeted funds be distributed through existing mechanisms within the Department of Health and Human Services and that funding be based on both technical merit and the priorities identified by the IOM.

4. Research and development conducted by organizations and groups committed to involving those who provide, purchase, insure, and receive care and to full and timely dissemination of the results.

5. National practice guidelines developed by professional organizations and groups committed to improving the rationality of the process, the validity of guidelines generated, and dissemination and education, thereby allowing the development of more effective quality assurance mechanisms.

6. The national organizations responsible for evaluating health care organizations (JCAHO, HCFA) should be required to base their

judgments in part on the effectiveness with which relevant research findings are integrated into health care organizations' day-to-day practice.

Demonstrable Openness and Objectivity

All phases of this National Quality Improvement Initiative must be characterized by objectivity and avoidance of conflict of interest; full and open engagement of those involved with and affected by health care; enough prestige to attract the participation of the "best" people; and a commitment to rapid, full and understandable presentation of results. This initiative, then, represents an effective public-private partnership that will best serve our nation's multiple interests.

CREATION OF A NATIONAL DATABASE

Throughout its analysis of the quality of the nation's health care, the Commission was frustrated by the lack of easily accessible, relevant data. The United States simply lacks the information it needs to understand the current level of the quality of care and to evaluate vigorously the effectiveness of national initiatives to improve quality. Today's lack of appropriateness and quality data is ironic given that many of us, physicians included, experience "information overload" in our day-to-day working lives. And the data that are available exist in a multiple of disparate databases, representing a microcosm of the state of medicine today: piecemeal and specialized, more artful than scientific, "high tech" but little analyzed.

Our frustration prompted consideration of the rapid creation of a national database, constructed around measures of the quality and appropriateness of care, not as a means toward *more* but *better* and *more scientific* information.[4]

Currently, as part of an Effectiveness Initiative proposed by the Health Care Financing Administration (HCFA) and being developed by the Department of Health and Human Services (HHS), the "Health Care Information Resource Center," (HCIRC) is under development. (7)

---

[4]The Commission approach had been stimulated by the ideas of Dr. Paul Ellwood, who calls for a program of "Outcomes Management," which includes an ongoing national database. (6)

HCFA proposed the HCIRC as a public-private collaboration to accomplish the following task:

- Provide the infrastructure (hardware and software for data communication, data storage, data management and processing for the creation and linkage of the shared data system) for the creation of analytic files; and to provide the resources for the assessment and use of analytic files by the center's participating organizations and other resources.
- Perform, on an ongoing basis, analysis to characterize the health status of populations, the persons receiving care, the care provided, the outcomes (mortality, morbidity, disability, expenditures) of care received, and initial assessments of the effectiveness of specific interventions.
- Identify the data needed to support the assessment of the effectiveness of health care interventions; and to define the formats and specifications for the acquisition and electronic transmission of such data.
- Assure the data integrity and protect the confidentiality of the data and the privacy of patients and providers.

Specifically, the Commission recommends that one or more respected organizations (e.g., IOM, JCAHO) be requested to undertake a detailed, 2–3 year examination which would: a) identify the data necessary to understand better the quality and appropriateness of health care; b) analyze the capability of current national, regional, state, and private databases to meet those needs; c) monitor progress on HHS's effort; and d) identify the technical feasibility, cost and value of creating a national database aimed at characterizing the quality and appropriateness of health care. Ultimately, the Commission would ideally like to see implemented, if feasible, a longitudinal database, where not only hospital data would be collected, but outpatient, ambulatory surgery, and long-term care data, as well.

Such information might be helpful as an aid to the development of practice guidelines. Along these lines, Dr. William Roper, administrator of the Health Care Financing Administration, stated in a recent issue of the *New England Journal of Medicine* that "Additional information is needed so that physicians can choose the most effective medical treatments. I believe that physicians are eager for such information and would use it readily. In the long run, better information about effectiveness should lead to better-documented standards of practice, which in turn should help reduce inappropriate care and lead to better quality." (8)

CONCLUSION

This National Quality Improvement Initiative is critical to the rational and effective use of our health care resources. It can and should be conducted through a public-private partnership that expands the work of many dedicated and experienced governmental agencies and private sector organizations. Each must be guided by well reasoned priorities and must use objective processes that engage all relevant parties. Over time, every important medical practice and technology could be carefully examined. Finally, using the stimulating power of existing external review mechanisms of government and the private sector, the results of such work will be rapidly integrated into day-to-day clinical practice and into the decisionmaking processes of health care organizations.

REFERENCES

1. Brook, R., and Kosecoff, J., "Competition and Quality," *Health Affairs* 7(3):150–161, Summer 1988, pp. 150–161.
2. Institute of Medicine, *Assessing Medical Technologies*, National Academy Press, Washington, DC, 1985.
3. Pellegrino, E., "The Most Humane Science: Some Notes on Liberal Education in Medicine and the University," *Bulletin of the Medical College of Virginia* 67(4):11–89, Summer, 1970.
4. Berwick, D., "Measuring and Maintaining Quality in a Health Maintenance Organization," *Quality of Care Technology Assessment: Report of a Forum of the Council on Health Care Technology,* Institute of Medicine, National Academy Press, Washington, DC, p. 33.
5. Roper, W., Winkenwerder, W., et al., "Effectiveness in Health Care: An Initiative to Evaluate and Improve Medical Practice," *NEJM* 319(18):1197–1202, November 3, 1988, p. 1197.
6. Ellwood, P., "Shattuck Lecture—Outcomes Management: A Technology of Patient Experience," *NEJM* 318(23):1549–1556, June 9, 1988.
7. Letter to Henry E. Simmons, The National Leadership Commission on Health Care, from Dr. Regina Phillips, HCFA, October 13, 1988.
8. Roper, W., "Perspectives on Physicians-Payment Reform," *NEJM* 319(13):865–867, September 29, 1988.

⌟ ⌞
Chapter Five
⌝ ⌜

Medical Professional Liability Reform

The Commission believes that the current system of malpractice litigation against providers of health care—hospitals, physicians and nurses—impedes the delivery of economical, high-quality care to American citizens. The Commission recognizes that patients should be fully compensated for injuries resulting from negligent care, and it supports strengthening procedures to identify and correct below-standard practices, but the present system of medical malpractice litigation does not achieve either goal and has other adverse consequences as well.

Exaggerated expectations by patients spawn many malpractice claims; the best medical care cannot always produce optimal outcomes. Highly publicized jury awards to malpractice plaintiffs tend to reinforce these unrealistic expectations. We must develop a discriminating medical malpractice system which compensates for truly negligent medical practice but not for simply a bad outcome.

Malpractice litigation has driven up the cost of medical care overall and, in some specialties, at a dramatic rate. Providers who can obtain malpractice insurance are forced to pass on its rising cost to patients (or third-party payers) through increased fees. For some providers (physicians, nurses and nurse mid-wives) in particular specialties or jurisdictions, malpractice insurance is simply not available at an affordable rate. We witness physicians refusing to perform risky procedures, changing location or specialties, or retiring early from medical practice. The lack of affordable insurance contributes to problems of recruiting and retaining nurses. The result has been loss of access to critical forms of medical care—such as obstetrics and complex surgical procedures—in many areas.

The fear of malpractice suits encourages defensive medicine, in which providers perform additional procedures, especially diagnostic ones, principally to protect themselves against law suits. Such procedures increase both the cost of care and sometimes health risks to patients. The rising rate of Cesarean section deliveries and excessive reliance on fetal monitoring are illustrations. Fear of suit also encourages providers to fail to record, or to withhold, detailed information about patient experience—information that can be critical in assessing treatment.

Both recipients and providers of medical care are hurt by indiscriminate malpractice suits—recipients because of increased costs, and providers because their professional reputations may be damaged by an unwarranted verdict. Indeed, recent declining medical and nursing school admissions have been linked to the adverse liability climate for health care providers.

The current system of malpractice litigation also corrodes the patient-physician relationship. We recognize that specialization and the increasing dependence on medical technology have exacted a toll, and members of the medical profession must make greater efforts, through direct personal dealings, to regain and keep the confidence of their patients. But the specter of malpractice suits also threatens the mutual confidence and trust essential to the healing process at work in the therapeutic relationship between patient and physician or nurse.

The problems of the current system of medical malpractice litigation—higher risks and costs, lessened access, and less mutual trust,—have been documented before. The Commission is concerned that, unless changed, the current system will impede essential reforms in the delivery and financing of medical care, such as the important changes, called for in this report, in the appropriateness and quality of care. Our proposed changes would discourage the excessive and sometimes imprudent, use of diagnostic and therapeutic techniques.

We are, therefore, convinced that the malpractice system must be reformed, and we are encouraged by the breadth of interest in reform both within the medical profession and outside it. Some promising proposals have been adopted experimentally on a state or local basis, and we strongly support continued exploration of potential solutions, and the adoption of the most promising reforms.

REFORM OF STATE MALPRACTICE LAW

Medical malpractice, like other forms of tort liability, is governed by state law, and several states have adopted new rules governing malpractice liability for specific types of injuries or designated treatment settings. We consider state reforms particularly important in four areas:

1. *Expert witnesses.* It is far too easy for a plaintiff to introduce the testimony, supposedly expert, of someone with no experience in the specialty of the defendant. Minimum criteria should be developed to establish the qualifications of an expert witness. There is also the danger that the "professional expert," who makes a living as a medical litigation consultant, will let his or her testimony be influenced by the desire to win or to enhance a personal reputation. Courts should probe for bias by allowing cross-examination as to how much of the expert witness's income comes from testifying in court. Professional societies could publish the names of expert witnesses and summaries of their testimony as a way of encouraging professional peer review.

2. *Standards of negligence.* Trial judges too often allow juries to infer negligence when the evidence shows merely a division in professional opinion about performance of a procedure. A finding of negligence should require evidence of a clear departure from a recognized standard of treatment, that is, treatment which a respectable body of experts support.

3. *Punitive damages.* They should be awarded only where there is convincing evidence of grave dereliction of professional responsibility or reckless departure from generally accepted standards of care. Damages should be used to compensate plaintiffs for injury, not punish defendants for misdeeds. Mere negligence should never be a basis for awarding punitive damages, and juries should be allowed to consider such damages only with the trial judge's approval and under his or her careful supervision. When punitive damages are awarded, they should go to the state, not the plaintiff.

4. *Contingency fees.* They serve a useful function by improving access to the courts for plaintiffs of modest means. But the mechanism is also open to abuse; it encourages a lottery mentality that frequently leads to litigating unwarranted claims. For this reason, the Commission supports some regulation of contingency fees, either through ceilings on contingency fees or through court review of such fees on a case-by-case basis.

Limitations on non-economic (or punitive) damages have been adopted in approximately twenty-five states, including California and Indiana. Another type of reform, perhaps more farsighted but less dramatic, is improving claims practices and litigation procedures. There are ways to reduce the excessive costs of our current system by improving claims handling by insurers, and reducing case preparation by both plaintiff and defense, through judicial encouragement of early settlement of claims. Speeding up the trial schedule for malpractice suits, a reform being adopted in North Carolina and Massachusetts, also holds great promise.

We think that other proposals currently under consideration also deserve further experimentation, such as periodic payments rather than lump sum damage awards, settlements providing payments over a plaintiff's lifetime and ending upon the death of the patient, reduced payments when other sources of funding are found, and limits on compensatory awards[1] paid to attorneys. States should also consider having judges or a knowledgeable triumvirate of arbitrators determine awards, rather than juries.

ALTERNATIVE SYSTEMS FOR ADJUDICATION OR COMPENSATION

A task force sponsored by the American Medical Association, 32 national medical specialty organizations, and the Council of Medical Specialty Societies (CMSS) has recently put forward a thoughtful proposal for a pilot project in the states. Its purpose is to reduce the cost of adjudicating malpractice claims, present them to triers of fact with the necessary expertise, and improve the distribution of compensation to all patients with meritorious claims. We support these goals and hope the AMA/ Specialty Society proposal will be tried out at the state level.

The Commission also supports other innovative approaches to alternative dispute resolution being tried in North Carolina and Wisconsin, such as arbitration, mediation, summary jury trials, and early neutral evaluation (similar to a *Special Master* in bankruptcy procedures). Malpractice litigation often ends in settlements on the courthouse steps, after lengthy trial preparation, so the long-range goal of removing this costly, complex litigation from the traditional courtroom environment could benefit all parties.

FEDERAL LEGISLATION

Although states are likely to be the major areas for serious reforms in malpractice litigation, we urge Congress to consider entering this field if

---

[1]We are aware of the concern that a proposal to limit the liability of physicians and institutions through caps on punitive and/or compensatory damages may adversely affect health industry manufacturers by exposing them to malpractice liability. States implementing such proposals should closely monitor their effects on health-related research and development by these manufacturers and others.

state reform efforts do not stem the tide of rising liability costs, which cause the havoc in health care described above.

Congress might consider a no-fault system which would compensate regardless of whether there has been malpractice. Such a no-fault proposal would have to be both affordable and efficient. Clearly, this idea deserves further study (like the Harvard Study under contract to New York State) and refinement. Special no-fault compensation funds could be adopted for particularly problematic areas of medical liability. Recent federal legislation has addressed the problem, for example, of vaccine-related injuries and has removed these troublesome cases from the tort system. A birth-related neurological injury fund might also be more effective at the national, rather than the state, level; the experience in Virginia and Florida with such a fund should be carefully watched carefully.[2]

Whatever precise reforms are adopted, we are convinced that the problem of malpractice must be addressed so that it does not impede solutions of the more critical issues confronting the health care system.

SELECTED BIBLIOGRAPHY

Litan, R., and Winston, C., editors, *Liability Perspectives and Policy*, The Brookings Institution, Washington, DC, 1988.

Medical Care and Medical Inquiries in the State of New York: A Pilot Study, Harvard Medical Practice Study Group, April 1987.

Medical Care and Medical Inquiries in the State of New York: An Interim Report, Harvard Medical Malpractice Study Group, March 1988.

Medical Malpractice: A Framework for Action, GAO/HRD-87-73, May 1987.

Medical Malpractice: No Agreement on the Problems or Solutions, GAO/HRD-86-50, February 1986.

Report of the Task Force on Medical Liability and Malpractice, U.S. Department of Health and Human Services, August 1987.

---

[2]Concerned about malpractice suits limiting access to obstetrical care, Virginia and Florida have both adopted laws which provide for the option of removing cases involving neurologic injuries to infants from the courts altogether. Instead, such cases are quickly heard in an administrative forum, and compensation is paid on a "no-fault" basis, regardless of physician negligence.

Chapter Six

Conclusion

The solutions proposed by the National Leadership Commission to the crises in the health care system call for systemic change to enable this country to achieve three principal goals: 1) an adequate level of care for all Americans, 2) a climate that fosters careful and effective cost control, and 3) significant, continual improvement in the quality of care. It will take time to achieve them, and the understanding and active participation of everyone who plays a major role in health care. Perhaps most importantly, achieving these goals will require a continuing campaign of public education to convince our compatriots that a healthy society is the responsibility of each one of us, as reflected in healthy lifestyles. The system-wide changes we propose depend on nation-wide cultural change.

The national health crisis is real. Our nation cannot call itself healthy if as many as one out of four Americans may lack adequate access to health care. Half of those, as many as 37 million Americans, lack any health insurance at all. And over 11 million of the uninsured are our children, the future of our society. If their ability to become productive citizens in our society is diminished, we are all diminished. Eleven million children without proper health care present us with a powerful mandate, one that the Commission has sought to respond to. Its strategy of providing access by asking every American to take responsibility for his or her own care and to assume a very small share of the cost of those who cannot assume that responsibility is eminently fair. It grows out of the same impulse of caring that led the country to provide social insurance to enable the elderly to live out their lives with dignity. A responsibility so widely shared is not an expensive burden for any one of us.

It never will become an expensive burden if we adopt an attitude about health care that encompasses an active understanding of the costs and benefits of our care, and the ability to negotiate fairly over the methods of treatment and their cost. By taking advantage of our federal system and using existing state agencies, plus a National Quality Improvement Initiative, both with significant cost-controlling potential, we will have a method for achieving that aim fairly and wisely.

In recent years, we have developed the research techniques to understand better the appropriateness and effectiveness of alternative procedures and to assure their efficient delivery. The solution to the problems in the quality of care is really quite simple. We had just never thought through a real investment strategy for quality health care before. This Commission has made that attempt, calling for a small increase in our investment in studying the appropriateness and effectiveness of the most common procedures we perform, learning better how to measure the performance of that care, and passing this information on in a coordinated fashion to physicians and patients. In a half-trillion dollar system, the amount of money to be spent is insignificant. The returns will be overwhelming both in terms of professional and patient confidence, in money saved on unnecessary and poor quality care, and in defusing the malpractice crisis that bedevils the health care system.

Believing in the need to provide access for all, understanding the difficulty of achieving cost control, and perceiving the deep uncertainty at the intellectual heart of medicine, the Commission is convinced that any solution in one part of the health care system must also relate to solutions in the other two parts. Certainly we want to provide access for all only to a system with effective cost control and the highest attainable quality. Therefore, we call for a solution in three parts to a system undermined by three problems. The problems are unnecessary, because we know how to solve them. They are larger than they ever needed to be because for years we understood them too little, we spent time blaming one party or another, and we did not have the scientific knowledge in some areas to respond to them. In recent years, we have found the will, we have learned that no one party is to blame, and we have developed the scientific ability to improve, to begin to close the gap between art and science that has characterized medicine for many years. There will always be some art and some uncertainty, because our science continuously stretches into new areas and because every patient presents a unique set of problems. But today we have some promising methods for reducing uncertainty. It is incumbent on us to use them and to improve them continually to advance the quality and control the cost of care.

We, as Commissioners, are dedicated to pursuing these solutions, presenting our strategies to the people who can take our suggestions and mold them into public policy, with the modifications that become necessary in the decisionmaking process. We understand that our strategy will need to be phased in over time. Demonstrations on the state or local level might point out ways to avoid the inevitable pitfalls that come with any change. Yet our vision of the future is clear; our understanding of the problems has deepened; our commitment to a system-wide solution is firm.

Above all, we are hopeful. Much has happened in just the two-and-a-half short years of the life of this Commission that indicates to us that all the parties involved in analyzing, delivering, paying for, and benefitting from health care in this country are anxious to become involved in a solution that works. We hope that our strategies will suggest a way.

⌐ ⌐
Technical Appendix I
⌐ ⌐

Financing Access to the Health Care System— Expenditures, Revenues, and Persons Covered

As noted in the report, the Commission recommends a shared responsibility for financing access to care for all Americans through a public-private partnership. To illustrate how this might be accomplished, the Commission designed a compromise proposal and developed some estimates of numbers and expenditures using the specific provisions of the proposal. These estimates and their underlying assumptions are provided here for the purpose of assisting public and private policy makers in the debate that will move our nation toward realizing the Commission's vision. The Commission makes no recommendations about the magnitudes of these estimates themselves or the assumptions made in their development.

COVERAGE AND BENEFITS UNDER THE UNIVERSAL ACCESS (UNAC) PROGRAM

As noted earlier, the Commission's plan would establish a program to provide health benefits to uninsured persons. This section presents estimates[1] of the following:

---

[1] The estimates presented in these analyses, and throughout this chapter, were developed using the Lewin/ICF Health Benefits Simulation Model (HBSM). The model is described in Appendix D. This model was supplemented by the Commission's assumptions.

1. the number of persons potentially affected by the Commission's plan;
2. the number of persons estimated to be covered under the program;
3. the total benefit costs for these persons under two illustrative benefit packages;
4. the impact of the inter-employer equity provisions of the Commission's plan on UNAC program expenditures; and
5. how the plan will affect benefit payments for existing public and private sources of payment for health care.

Number of Persons Potentially Affected by the Commission's Plan

The plan proposed by the Commission was designed to encourage everyone to have his or her own insurance coverage and to provide an incentive to employers to offer insurance coverage for a basic level of care. It was also designed to make the process fairer between employers, easing the burden on those companies who foot the health care bill for spouses who could be covered by their own employers, but choose not to be, usually because their plan is less generous.

In this section, the number of persons who have any potential at all of being affected by the Commission's plan is estimated. Private and public sector charges are included in the figures. In the next section, the number of those actually expected to have coverage through the program is estimated. As with any estimates, a number of assumptions had to be made that would likely change along with even minor changes in specific provisions of this illustrative proposal.

The Commission's proposed plan potentially could affect the sources and levels of health coverage for over half of all Americans. As shown in Table 1, the plan potentially could change the source of health coverage and/or level of health coverage for about 125.8 million persons. This includes the estimated 37.4 million persons who are currently uninsured and the 22.1 million persons covered by Medicaid under current law.[2] In addition, it was estimated that about 19.5 million individuals would drop their non-group coverage to become covered under either: 1)

---

[2]This study assumes that some form of Medicaid would be retained for persons in nursing homes. Nursing home residents currently covered by Medicaid are excluded from our estimates of the number of persons potentially covered under the fund.

newly established employer plans, or 2) UNAC. These 19.5 million persons are likely to drop their non-group coverage, because the employer-financed plan (including the individual's share of costs) would be less expensive to the individual than the non-group coverage. It is likely that some of these individuals will supplement the benefits provided by an employer plan or the UNAC program with additional individual coverage.

The 125.8 million persons potentially affected by the Commission's plan also include 26.6 million persons whose source of coverage potentially could change due to the "inter-employer equity" provisions of the

Table 1: Persons Whose Health Coverage Would Be Potentially Affected by the Commission's Proposed Plan by Insured Status Under Current Law in 1988 (in millions)

	Persons
Uninsured under current law[a]	37.4
Insured by Medicaid under current law[b]	22.1
Insured through non-group insurance under current law	19.5
Inter-employer equity provisions	26.6
Workers insured as dependents under current law[c]	[21.5]
Children allocated to program[d]	[5.1]
Workers and dependents covered under existing employer plans potentially covered by program[e]	1.9
Workers and dependents affected by minimum benefits and employer contribution standards[f]	18.3
Total potentially affected by Commission's plan	125.8

Source: Lewin/ICF estimates using the Health Benefits Simulation Model (HBSM).

[a]There are about 1.9 million early retirees, about 136,000 of whom are uninsured. These uninsured early retirees are included among the 37.4 million uninsured.

[b]Includes only those covered by Medicaid for acute care. We assume the Medicaid program continues for persons receiving long-term care.

[c]Includes working spouses who might become covered under either the UNAC program or their own employer's plan if offered.

[d]Includes children allocated to either another employer's plan or the UNAC program due to provisions requiring that dependent children be picked up by one parent's plan in cases where both parents are employed.

[e]Firms that currently offer coverage whose average wage and salary payment per employee is below 250 percent of the poverty level for a single individual (about $14,000 in 1988) might elect to discontinue their plan and cover these workers and dependents under the program by paying the X_1 fee.

[f]We estimate that there are about 19.5 million workers and dependents who are covered by employer plans which fall short of the minimum benefit and employer contribution standards. Of these 19.5 million persons, 1.2 million are counted among the 1.9 million persons whose employer could terminate their plan and cover their workers under the program by paying the X_1 fee.

plan. These persons include about 21.5 million workers who were covered under their spouse's employer plan under current law who would become covered under either their own employer's plan or the UNAC program due to the elimination of spousal waivers. The 26.6 million persons affected by the inter-employer equity provisions also include about 5.1 million children in families with two working parents who would be affected by the provision which requires one of the parents' employers to cover the children. However, employers may continue to cover working dependent spouses or provide wraparound coverage. To the extent this occurs, the number of persons actually affected by the inter-employer equity provisions could be substantially less than 26.6 million.

Many persons who are currently covered under an employer health plan also will be affected. About 3.9 million of the 125.8 million persons affected by the Commission's plan would be part-time workers and their dependents who are employed by a firm which offers a health plan but limits eligibility to full-time workers.[3] Also, about 18.3 million workers and dependents are covered under an existing employer plan which falls short of the minimum benefit and employer contribution requirements of the Commission's proposal.

Some persons who are currently insured by an existing employer health plan could become covered under the UNAC program. This is because under the Commission's plan, we expect almost all firms with *average* wages and salaries per employee equal to or above 250 percent of the poverty level for a single individual ($14,000 in 1988) would provide coverage for basic level of care.[4] Those firms with *average* wages and salaries per employee below 250 percent of poverty may choose between offering coverage or covering their workers under the UNAC program by paying the X_1 fee and terminating their existing plan.[5] However, few of the employers who currently offer health benefits have an average payroll as low as $14,000 per worker. We estimate that of the 138 million Americans covered by employer health plans, there are only about 1.9

---

[3]It is estimated in this analysis that there are about 3.0 million part-time workers age 18 or older who are employed by a firm which limits coverage to full-time workers. It is further estimated that these workers have about 900,000 dependent children. Under current policy these 3.9 million persons are either currently insured by Medicaid, covered under non-group plans, or completely without insurance.

[4]This assumption was specified by the Commission.

[5]For purposes of comparison with the $14,000 standard, average annual payroll is defined as total annual wages and salaries before payroll deductions divided by the average number of workers per week, including full-time and part-time workers, employed by the firm during the year.

million workers and dependents who are in plans sponsored by firms with average salaries below this level.[6] Under the Commission's plan, all of these individuals potentially could become covered under the UNAC program.

Estimate of Number of Persons Covered Under the UNAC Program

As shown in Table 2, of the 125.8 million persons potentially affected by the Commission's plan, the most reasonable estimate is that about 67.9 million will become covered under the UNAC program. Another 32.6 million persons will become covered under plans established by employers in response to the Commission's proposal. The remaining 25.3 million of the 125.8 million persons potentially affected by the Commission's plan are persons who would be covered under existing employer plans. Most of these 25.3 million people would be persons in plans which must improve to meet the minimum benefit and employer contribution standards of the Commission's plan. If all employers chose to provide insurance rather than pay the X_1 fee, the number could be as small as 42.9 million.[7]

The estimates of the number of persons covered under the UNAC program are based upon several key assumptions. First, it is assumed that all employers who do not now provide insurance and whose average payroll is more than 250 percent of the poverty level for a single individual (approximately $14,000 in 1988) will offer insurance. The rationale for this assumption is that, on average, the X_1 fee payment for firms below this payroll standard will be about two-thirds of what they would pay for insurance (the costs to firms of paying the X_1 fee vis-à-vis purchasing insurance are discussed in Technical Appendix II). Based upon this assumption, it is estimated that about 34.1 million of the estimated 67.3 million full-time workers (i.e., those who work 25 hours or

---

[6]The number of persons in existing plans who potentially could be moved from employer coverage to the program is very sensitive to the average salary standard chosen. For example, we estimate that if the average salary standard were increased to $17,000 (i.e., 300 percent of poverty) the number of persons potentially transferred to the fund would increase from about 1.9 million persons to about 10.6 million.

[7]This is a very rough estimate, including: 6.9 of 37.4 million uninsured (the uninsured non-workers who are not dependents of workers); 21 of 22.1 million Medicaid recipients; 2.7 of 19.5 million non-group insurance beneficiaries (who do not work); and 12.3 million uninsured part-year workers (who would be in the program part of the year and in an employer plan part of the year).

Table 2: Persons Potentially Affected by the Commission's Plan by Source of Coverage upon Implementation (in millions)

	Persons Potentially Affected	Estimated Allocation of Affected Persons by Source of Coverage		
		Covered Under Existing Employer Plan	Covered Under Newly Established Employer Plan	Covered Under Program
Uninsured under current law[a]	37.4	1.6[b]	9.7	26.1
Insured by Medicaid under current law[c]	22.1		1.3	20.8
Insured through non-group insurance under current law	19.5		14.8	4.7
Inter-employer equity provisions	26.6	4.7	6.8	15.1
Workers insured as dependents under current law[d]	[21.5][e]	[3.8]	[5.5]	[12.2]
Children allocated to program[f]	[5.1]	[0.9]	[1.3]	[2.9]
Workers and dependents covered under existing employer plans potentially covered by UNAC program[g]	1.9	0.7		1.2
Workers and dependents affected by minimum benefits and employer contribution standards[h]	18.3	18.3		
Total	125.8	25.3	32.6	67.9

Source: Lewin/ICF estimates using the Health Benefits Simulation Model (HBSM).

[a] There are about 1.9 million early retirees, about 136,000 of whom are uninsured. These uninsured early retirees are included among the 37.4 million uninsured.

[b] We estimate there are about 1.6 million dependents of covered workers who are not covered because the covered worker declined the family coverage option. We assume that all employees elect the family coverage option to avoid paying the X_2 fee.

[c] Includes only those covered by Medicaid for acute care. It is assumed that the Medicaid program continues for persons receiving long-term care.

[d] Includes working spouses who might become covered under either their own employer's plan if offered or the UNAC program.

[e] There are about 21.5 million workers covered as dependents on their spouse's plan. Of these about 3.8 million had declined coverage under their own employer's plan. We assumed that all of these 3.8 million dependents would take coverage under their own employer's plan to avoid paying the X_2 fee. The remaining 17.7 million are working for an employer who does not offer coverage. Of these, about 6.6 million are part-time workers, all of whom would become covered under the fund and about 11.1 million are full-time workers. Of those who are full-time workers, we assume that 5.5 million will become covered under a newly established plan and 5.6 million will become covered under the program.

[f] Includes children allocated to either another employer's plan or the program due to provisions requiring that dependent children be picked up by one parent's plan in cases where both parents are employed.

[g] Firms that currently offer coverage whose average wage and salary payment per employee is below 250 percent of the poverty level for a single individual (about $14,000 in 1988) may discontinue their plan and cover these workers and dependents under the program by paying the X_1 fee.

[h] We estimate that there are about 19.5 million workers and dependents who are covered by employer plans which fall short of the minimum benefit and employer contribution standards. Of these 19.5 million persons, 1.2 million are counted among the 1.9 million persons whose employer could terminate their plan and cover their workers under the program by paying the X_1 fee.

more per week) and dependents in firms that do not offer insurance will become covered under UNAC.[8]

A second key assumption is that all employers who do not cover part-time workers (i.e., persons working less than 25 hours per week) will choose to cover these workers under UNAC by paying the X_1 fee rather than providing insurance. The rationale for this assumption is that the X_1 fee employers will pay for part-time workers on average will be less than half of the cost of providing insurance to these workers. Based on this assumption, we estimate that about 12.2 million part-time workers and their dependents will become covered under the program. Of these, about 3.9 million are part-time workers and their dependents who currently work for a firm which offers insurance but limits coverage to full-time workers.

A third key assumption is that among firms which currently offer insurance, employers eligible to participate in the program will choose to terminate existing plans and cover workers under the program only in instances where the existing plan falls short of the minimum benefit and employer contribution standards. The rationale for this assumption is that firms facing the added cost of complying with these provisions will be more inclined than other employers to cover workers under the program. However, most firms that currently offer benefits exceeding these standards are more likely to retain these benefits rather than shifting their employees to the less comprehensive coverage provided by the program.

As shown in Table 2, about 1.9 million persons are covered by existing employer plans sponsored by firms which could decide it would be economical to cover their employees under the fund by paying the X_1 fee (i.e., the average payroll per worker falls below 250 percent of poverty). Of these, about 1.2 million persons are in plans which also fall short of the minimum benefit and employer contribution standards. It is assumed that all 1.2 million of these persons will become covered under the program while persons covered by plans that exceed these standards will remain covered under the employers' plan.

It is also assumed that all employers will elect not to cover working dependent spouses. However, under the Commission's plan, employers will have the option of extending coverage to working spouses if they choose to do so or provide wraparound coverage. Yet, employers are unlikely to choose this option, because they will now be paying the Y

---

[8]The 67.3 million full-time workers and dependents whose employers do not provide insurance includes about 45 million persons who are covered by other sources such as Medicaid, non-group policies, and as dependents on their spouse's plan. About 27.3 million of these persons are currently without any form of insurance.

premium to share in the costs for all poor people and perhaps the X_1 fees on part-time workers. It is likely that most employers will be eager to offset these increases in business expenses with reductions in other employee benefits, such as providing full family coverage. Also, if employers do extend coverage to working spouses, the benefits will most likely be in the form of a supplement to coverage provided under the program rather than a substitute for the program as primary payer. Supplemental coverage of this type would have no impact on expenditures under the program.

Finally, the number of persons who are covered under the UNAC program could be substantially smaller than 67.9 million depending upon: 1) the number of employers who respond to the X_1 fee by providing health coverage rather than paying the fee and 2) the number of employers who extend coverage to working dependent spouses. The number of persons covered under the program could also be larger than 67.9 million if all employers who fall below the average payroll standard terminate their plans and elect to pay the X_1 fee instead.

Benefit Costs Under the UNAC Program

To develop illustrative estimates of the cost of the plan, the impact of two prototype benefit packages was estimated. These packages are only illustrative; they were used solely for the purpose of analysis. They do **not** represent Commission recommendations for a national package of benefits, since the Commission has decided not to recommend specific services to be included.[9] The Commission recommends that the national package provide a range of services, including preventive and mental health care. The first, "basic-option" plan provides a package of benefits which represents a typical or "average cost" employer plan. The second illustrative plan, the "low-option" plan, provides a more limited level of coverage, placing emphasis on preventive care rather than catastrophic health coverage. These benefit packages, the provisions of which are described in Appendix B, are:

> The **basic-option** illustrative benefits package, which would cover hospital care (30 day maximum for mental health hospitalizations), physician services (excluding general check-ups and well-baby care), drugs, mental health care (up to 50 visits), and outpatient care. The plan would have an annual deductible of $100 per person with a 20 percent copayment by the beneficiary for expenses over

---

[9]Instead, the Commission recommends an ongoing mechanism for updating the national basic package of services. See chapter 2 for more information.

the deductible. (There would be no separate deductible for families.) There would be a limit of $1,000 on annual cost sharing per person ($3,000 per family).

The **low-option** illustrative benefits package would provide a basic level of services which emphasizes primary and preventive care rather than catastrophic coverage. The plan would cover inpatient hospital care (14 day maximum), outpatient services, prescription drugs, and well baby care. Neither dental nor mental health care would be covered. The plan would have a $50 deductible per person ($150 per family) with no coinsurance. There would be no limit on annual cost sharing.[10]

Table 3 presents the average annual premium under these two plans for family and individual coverage. These premium estimates reflect the unique demographic composition of the population that would be covered under the program. On average, the persons covered under the program are younger than the currently insured population, and a disproportionate share are male, low income, and non-white. These estimates also reflect that the inter-employer equity provisions of the plan will tend to reduce the average number of persons covered under the family coverage option, because children are allocated to one or the other employer plans in families with two working spouses.

If the basic-option plan were implemented in 1988, it is estimated that the benefits provided by the program, **excluding** administrative costs, would be about $76.2 billion. As shown in Table 4, under the basic-option plan, these expenditures include about $54.9 billion in ben-

Table 3: Average Annual Premium Under Illustrative Plans for Individual and Family Coverage in 1988[a]

	Basic-option Benefits Package	Low-option Benefits Package
Individual coverage	$1,100	$920
Family coverage	$2,270	$2,170

Source: Lewin/ICF estimates.

[a]Estimates reflect the assumption that administrative costs under the plan will be about 8 percent of benefit payments. Premium estimates are for workers and dependents potentially covered under the fund.

---

[10]A low-cost plan could be designed which places greater emphasis on covering catastrophic expenses by increasing the number of hospital days covered. The cost of such a plan could be reduced by increasing cost-sharing provisions (deductibles and coinsurance).

Table 4: Total Expenditures Under Commission's UNAC Program Fund (in billions of 1988 dollars)[a]

	Basic-option Plan		Low-option Plan	
	Total Benefits Under Plan	Total Benefits Plus Administration[b]	Total Benefits Under Plan	Total Benefits Plus Administration[b]
Employees and dependents	$35.7	$38.6	$32.3	$34.9
Below 150 percent of poverty line	[16.4]	[17.8]	[14.9]	[16.1]
Above 150 percent of poverty line	[19.3]	[20.8]	[17.4]	[18.8]
Non-workers	40.5	43.7	37.8	40.8
Total	$76.2	$82.3	$70.1	$75.7

Source: Lewin/ICF estimates.

[a]These estimates were developed using the Lewin/ICF Health Benefits Simulation Model described in Appendix A.

[b]It is assumed that administrative expenses for the plan will be about 8 percent of benefit payments.

efits to workers and dependents. As shown in Table 4, under the basic-option plan these expenditures include about $35.7 billion in benefits to workers and dependents. About $16.4 billion of these expenditures would be for workers and dependents with incomes below 150 percent of the official poverty threshold.[11] The fund would provide about $40.5 billion in benefits to non-workers.[12]

Total benefit payments under the low-option plan would be about $70.1 billion. As shown in Table 4, about $32.3 billion of these expenditures would be for workers and dependents while about $37.8 billion would be for non-workers. Benefit payments to workers and dependents with incomes below 150 percent of the poverty line would be about $14.9 billion under the low-option plan.

As shown in Table 4, total costs for the UNAC program, including

[11]The poverty threshold for a family of four was about $11,170 in 1988.

[12]These benefit payment estimates reflect that the demographic composition of the uninsured population differs considerably from that of the insured population and that their utilization of health expenditures differs accordingly. The uninsured tend to be younger than the general population, and a disproportionate share are males and low-income minorities.

benefit payments and administrative expenses, would be about $82.3 billion under the basic-option plan and about $75.7 billion under the low-option plan. For the basic-option plan this includes $76.2 billion in benefits payments and about $6.1 billion in administrative expenses. For the low-option plan this includes $70.1 billion in benefit payments and about $5.6 billion in administrative costs.

Administration costs for the program were assumed to be equal to about 8 percent of benefit payments. This is the nationwide average of administrative costs for all private insurers.[13] Program expenditures could be higher or lower due to cost control measures and the guidelines on quality and appropriateness/effectiveness of care resulting from the research proposed under the Commission's plan. The potential savings from appropriateness/effectiveness research are discussed in Technical Appendix III.

Impact of Inter-Employer Equity Provisions

The benefit payment estimates presented in Table 4 reflect the impact of provisions in the Commission's plan which would promote inter-employer equity. These provisions would: 1) give working spouses the option of accepting coverage on their own job, or accepting wraparound coverage from their spouse's employer and 2) have one of the employer's plans pick up dependent children in families with two working parents.[14] These provisions are intended to distribute the cost of insuring dependents more equitably across employers. This will tend to offset current practice by shifting the cost of insuring workers and their dependents away from industries where coverage levels are high (i.e., manufacturing and finance) to industries where coverage levels are comparatively low (i.e., services and trade).

Table 5 shows the impact of these inter-employer equity provisions on benefit payments under the Commission's plan. Under the basic-option benefits package, these provisions would account for about $15.8 billion of the $76.2 billion in benefit payments under the Commission's plan. Under the low-option package, these provisions would account for about $14.2 billion of the $70.1 billion in benefit payments under the plan. If these inter-employer equity provisions were eliminated from the Commission's plan, total benefit payments under the program would drop to $60.4 billion under the basic-option benefits package and about $55.9 billion under the low-option benefits package.

---

[13]This estimate is based on Health Care Financing Administration (HCFA) data reported in the National Health Accounts.

[14]These assumptions were specified by the Commission.

Table 5: Benefit Payments Under the Commission's Plan With and Without the Inter-employer Equity Provisions in 1988 (in billions of dollars)

	Basic-option Benefits Package	Low-option Benefits Package
Total benefit payments	$76.2	$70.1
Payments attributed to inter-employer equity provisions	(15.8)	(14.2)
Total benefit payments without inter-employer equity provisions	$60.4	$55.9

Source: Lewin/ICF estimates.

In response to a concern that the inter-employer equity provisions could shift some individuals out of generous employer plans into plans which are less comprehensive, the Commission's plan permits employers to offer coverage to working spouses if they choose to do so. This option will permit employers and employees to negotiate benefits packages which best meet the needs of the firm's work force. To the extent this occurs, it could substantially reduce expenditures under UNAC. This approach also permits a more equitable distribution of health care costs across employers without imposing potentially catastrophic hardships on households.

As an alternative to offering standard coverage to working spouses, many employers may elect to offer a secondary coverage option for dependents who are covered under another plan. Under this arrangement, each employer would be the primary payer for care provided to employees and dependent children allocated to that plan. The secondary coverage option provided by the other working parent's employer would then be secondary payer for services consumed by these individuals. However, because the spouse's employer plan remains the primary payer, these secondary coverage plans will have little impact on program expenditures.

Impact on Health Expenditures by Source of Payment

As discussed above, in addition to the UNAC program created under the Commission's plan, many employers will be required to establish health plans of their own. For many individuals, existing sources of payment for care will be replaced by either the UNAC program or these newly established plans. Also, the Commission's proposals are estimated to

induce an increase in public and private health care expenditures combined of between $14 and $16 billion as health coverage is extended to the
uninsured.

Table 6 presents total benefit payments under the basic-option and
low-option plans by the source of payment for health expenditures under current law. Total benefit payments by newly established employer
plans will be about $19.2 billion under the basic-option benefits package
and about $17.4 billion under the low-option benefits package. By com-
parison, total benefit payments under the program will be about $76.2
billion under the basic-option plan and about $70.1 billion under the low-
option plan.

Of the $76.2 billion in total UNAC program benefit payments under
the basic-option plan, about $28.4 billion would cover services currently
financed by Medicaid.[15] Another $4.8 billion of fund expenditures would
have been covered by other welfare and county hospitals under current
law. About $4.5 billion would be expenditures that are currently in the
form of charity care by providers (primarily hospitals).

As shown in Table 6, under the basic-option plan about $12.2 bil-
lion of benefits provided under the program would be expenditures for
working dependents who would have been covered under their spouse's
plan under current law.[16] Another $3.6 billion would be expenditures for
dependent children who under current law would have been covered
under an existing employer plan. Another $2.1 billion of UNAC program
expenditures are those that would have been paid through individual
non-group insurance under current law (as discussed above, it was assumed that eligible individuals drop their non-group insurance—most
to become covered by plans established by firms and some under the
program). About $7.6 billion of the expenditures covered under the pro-
gram would have been paid out-of-pocket by households under current
law.

About $13.0 billion of program expenditures under the basic-option
plan will be attributed to increases in health care utilization induced by
the greater availability of health insurance.[17] To estimate induced de-

---

[15]This estimate excludes the cost of nursing home care for institutionalized. It is assumed that Medicaid would continue to provide coverage to the nursing home population
as under current law.

[16]As noted earlier, this amount could be much smaller if the employer of the husband
behaves differently from the assumption and continues to cover the wife. ("Husband" and
"wife" are used here to clarify the example.)

[17]These estimated increases in utilization may overstate the utilization induced by the
plan for two reasons. First, many persons who currently lack insurance may be individuals
who are disinclined to consume health care regardless of their insured status for various
cultural and/or behavioral reasons. Second, the increase in utilization is likely to be miti-
gated by cost containment efforts under the Commission's plan.

mand, it was assumed that as coverage is extended to the uninsured, their utilization of health services covered under the program will increase to the level of insured persons within the same age, sex, income, and health status groups (the utilization response estimates are discussed in greater detail in Appendix A). Under the basic-option plan, this enhanced utilization will result in an increase in total health expenditures of about $24.4 billion of which about $16.0 billion would be covered by either the program ($13.0 billion) or newly established employer plans ($3.0 billion). The remaining $8.4 billion would be paid out-of-pocket by households according to the plan's cost sharing provisions. Under the low-option plan, the total increase in health expenditures will be about $21.9 billion, of which about $14.1 billion would be covered by either the program ($11.5 billion) or newly established employer plans ($2.6 billion).

PLAN FINANCING OPTIONS

The Commission proposes to finance expenditures under the UNAC program with a combination of fees from employers and employees. This section describes these fees and provides estimates of the rates necessary to finance the benefits provided under the Commission's plan. Also examined are alternative funding options and estimated rates required to finance the health services research proposed under the Commission's plan.

Fee Base and Revenue Requirements

Tables 6 and 7 show how expenditures under the program, including benefit payments and administrative costs, would be financed under the Commission's plan for the basic-option benefits package. The Commission's plan would finance the cost of insuring non-workers and workers and dependents with incomes **below** 150 percent of the poverty threshold ($61.5 billion) with: 1) state and Federal revenues that would have been expended under the Medicaid program under current policy, and 2) a premium from employers and individuals known as the Y health insurance premium. In 1988, state and Federal expenditures for acute care (i.e., non-nursing home care) under the Medicaid program, including benefit payments and administrative costs, would be about $32.5 billion.[18] Of this $32.5 billion in Medicaid expenditures, about $18.2 bil-

---

[18]These estimates exclude Medicaid expenditures for nursing home care. In this analysis it is assumed that the Medicaid program is restructured only for acute care (i.e., non-nursing home care) and that the Medicaid program is retained in some form to cover long-term care.

Table 6: Total Benefits Paid Under the UNAC Program by Source of Payment for These Expenditures Under Current Law (in billions of 1988 dollars)

	Basic-option			Low-option		
	All Benefits	Plans Established by Firms	UNAC	All Benefits	Plans Established by Firms	UNAC
Expenses covered by Medicaid under current law[a]	$30.2	$1.8	$28.4	$30.2	$1.8	$28.4
Expenses for working dependents covered under their spouse's plan under current law	16.0	3.8	12.2	14.2	3.3	10.9
Expenses for dependent children	4.7	1.1	3.6	4.3	1.0	3.3
Expenses paid through charity care under current law[b]	5.7	1.2	4.5	5.3	1.1	4.2
Expenses paid through other welfare and county hospitals	5.8	1.0	4.8	4.4	0.7	3.7
Expenses paid through non-group insurance under current law[c]	7.9	5.8	2.1	7.9	5.8	2.1
Expenses paid out-of-pocket by households under current law	9.1	1.5	7.6	7.1	1.1	6.0
Expenditures induced by the availability of insurance (induced demand)	16.0[d]	3.0	13.0	14.1[e]	2.6	11.5
Total benefit payments under program	$95.4	$19.2	$76.2	$87.5	$17.4	$70.1

Source: Lewin/ICF estimates.

[a]Includes only Medicaid expenditures for the non-institutionalized. It is assumed that Medicaid coverage would continue for nursing home residents.

[b]Based on AHA data on bad debt and charity care in 1986. Total uncompensated care in 1988 is estimated to be about $8.1 billion. The AHA estimates that about 70 percent of this is attributed to the uninsured.

[c]In this analysis we assumed that individuals who currently purchase individual non-group insurance will drop the non-group insurance and accept coverage under either the UNAC program or newly established plans.

[d]Under the basic-option plan, total health care expenditures induced by the availability of insurance were $24.4 billion. Due to the cost sharing provisions of the basic-option plan about $8.4 billion would be paid by households out-of-pocket with $16.0 billion paid either by newly established plans or by the program.

[e]Under the low-option plan, total health care expenditures induced by the availability of insurance would be $21.9 billion, about $14.1 billion of which would be paid either by newly established plans or by the program.

lion were paid by the Federal government and about $14.3 billion were paid by the states.[19] Under the Commission's plan, all of these monies would be transferred to the fund for the program.[20]

Thus, of the $61.5 billion needed to insure non-workers and workers and dependents below 150 percent of the poverty line, about $32.5 billion would be financed with state and Federal funds, and about $29.0 billion would be financed with the Y premium. The Commission's plan would allocate the cost of raising these $29.0 billion in Y premium revenues equally across employers and on individuals. Under this formula, the Y premiums on employers and employees would each raise revenues of about $14.5 billion.

The Commission's plan would allocate the cost of insuring workers and dependents with incomes *above* 150 percent of the poverty line ($20.8 billion), so that 80 percent of the costs are financed by the X_1 fee on employers, and 20 percent are financed by the X_2 fee on individuals. Under this formula, the X_1 fee would have to raise $16.6 billion, and the X_2 fee would have to raise about $4.2 billion. Table 8 presents the sources and uses of funds under the low-option benefits package.

The bases for the Y premium and X fees are defined as follows:

Y Premium used to fund insurance for non-workers and workers and dependents below 150 percent of the poverty line, without insurance:

> **Employer Base**: The Y premium is a payroll fee applied to all wages and salaries for all workers on the employer's payroll up to the Social Security maximum covered earnings level ($45,000 in 1988).

> **Individual Base**: The Y premium on families applies to adjusted gross income over 150 percent of the poverty level up to the Social Security maximum for covered earnings.

X Fee used to fund insurance for workers and dependents with incomes above the poverty line, without insurance:

> **Employer Base for X_1 Fee:** The X_1 fee is paid by the employers on all non-covered workers up to the Social Security maximum covered earnings level.

---

[19]State expenditures for Medicaid are matched with a Federal contribution. The Federal Medicaid matching rate varies by state. Nationwide, about 56 percent of Medicaid expenditures are paid by the Federal government.

[20]As explained above, the UNAC program would cover all persons currently covered by Medicaid, except nursing home residents, and the Medicaid program would be restructured for non-nursing home care.

Table 7: Sources and Uses of Funds Under UNAC Basic-option Benefits Package (in billions of 1988 dollars)[a]

| | | Uses of Funds | | |
| | | | Costs of Insuring Workers and Dependents | |
Sources of Funds	*Total*	*Cost of Insuring Non-Workers*	*Below 150 Percent of Poverty*	*Above 150 Percent of Poverty*
Government contributions[b]				
Federal government	$18.2	$17.1	$1.1	
State governments	14.3	13.5	0.8	
Employer fees				
Y premium on wages and salaries for all workers up to $45,000	14.4	6.5	7.9	
X_1 fee on payroll wages and salaries up to $45,000 for all workers in plans that do not offer coverage	16.6			16.6
Individual fees				
Y premium on adjusted gross income above 150 percent of the poverty line up to $45,000	14.4	6.5	7.9	
X_2 premium on adjusted gross income above 150 percent of the poverty line up to $45,000 for non-covered persons	4.2			4.2
Total[c]	$82.3	$43.7	$17.8	$20.8

Source: Lewin/ICF estimates using the Health Benefits Simulation Model.
[a]Estimates include administrative costs.
[b]Includes state and federal Medicaid expenditures for acute care (i.e., excludes long-term care) under current law.
[c]Components may not sum to totals due to rounding.

Table 8: Sources and Uses of Funds Under UNAC Low-option Benefits Package (in billions of 1988 dollars)[a]

Sources of Funds	Uses of Funds			
	Total	Cost of Insuring Non-Workers	Costs of Insuring Workers and Dependents	
			Below 150 Percent of Poverty	Above 150 Percent of Poverty
Government contributions[b]				
Federal government	$18.2	$17.1	$1.1	
State governments	14.3	13.5	0.8	
Employer fees				
Y premium on wages and salaries for all workers up to $45,000	12.2	5.1	7.1	
X_1 fee on payroll wages and salaries up to $45,000 for all workers in plans that do not offer coverage	15.0			15.0
Individual fees				
Y premium on adjusted gross income above the poverty line up to $45,000	12.2	5.1	7.1	
X_2 fee on adjusted gross income above the poverty line up to $45,000 for non-covered persons	3.8			3.8
Total[c]	$75.7	$40.8	$16.1	$18.8

Source: Lewin/ICF estimates using the Health Benefits Simulation Model.
[a]Estimates include administrative costs.
[b]Includes state and federal Medicaid expenditures for acute care (i.e., excludes long-term care) under current law.
[c]Components may not sum to totals due to rounding.

Individual Base for X₂ Fee: The X_2 tax is fee paid on adjusted gross income over 150 percent of the poverty level up to the Social Security maximum covered earnings level for uninsured persons.

Both the Y and X_2 fees on individuals are applied to the amount of adjusted gross income **over** 150 percent of the poverty level.

Fee Preferences

The X_1 and X_2 fees would be structured so that certain groups of firms and individuals would pay fees at preferential rates. These preferences include:

New Business: The X_1 fee for firms that do not provide health insurance would be reduced for firms in existence three years or less. The X_1 fee would be reduced by 60 percent for firms up to one year of age, 40 percent for firms up to two years of age, and 20 percent for firms up to 3 years of age. The full amount of the X_1 fee would be paid by firms over three years of age. The X_2 fee for employees of those businesses would remain the same.

Self-Employed Persons: Self-employed persons who do not have health insurance will be required to pay both the X_1 and the X_2 fees. To relieve the burden on this group of workers, the Commission proposes to reduce the combined fee by the same proportion that the social security FICA rate is reduced for self-employed persons (FICA for self-employed persons is about 86.7 percent of the combined employer/employee contribution for wage and salary workers).

Small Firms: The X_1 fee for small firms (5 or fewer employees) that do not provide health insurance would be reduced by about 20 percent.

Part-Time Workers: The X_1 and X_2 fee rates would be scaled downward for part-time workers in proportion to the number of hours worked per week. For purposes of determining the amount of this fee preference, part-time workers are defined as persons working less than 35 hours per week.[21] For part-time workers, the X_1 and X_2

---

[21]Note that for purposes of scaling down the X_1 and X_2 fee rates for part-time workers, part-time worker is defined as an employee working less than 35 hours per week. This differs from the definition of part-time used in determining whether an employer may cover the worker under the program which is currently set at 25 hours per week.

fee rates would be computed as the standard fee rates reduced by the proportion of the week they usually work. The purpose of this provision is to prevent the X_1 fee from discouraging employment of part-time workers and to lessen the X_2 fee burden on part-time workers who typically have low incomes.

In this analysis, it is assumed that these preferences would be achieved by exempting a portion of the revenue base from the fee for those groups selected for preferential treatment. A uniform rate would then be applied to this new, effective revenue base. This approach permits the convenience of working with a single rate while achieving the desired relief for self-employed persons, small businesses, and new businesses. Table 8 presents the bases for the X and Y fees and the effective bases for these fees after adjustment for preferences.

Required Fee Rates

Estimates of the effective revenue base for each fee and the revenue which must be raised from each of these sources are shown in Table 10 (the revenue requirements for each fee are taken from the sources and uses of funds analysis shown in Tables 7 and 8). In 1988, the effective Y premium base for employers would be about $2.1 trillion, while the effective Y base for employees, which includes the amount of adjusted gross income over 150 percent of the poverty level up to the Social Security covered earnings level for all taxpayers, would be about $2.2 trillion. The Y fee base for individuals is larger than the Y fee base for employers because 1) the Y fee base for individuals includes incomes of both workers and non-workers while the Y fee base for employers includes only workers, and 2) the Y fee base for individuals is based upon adjusted gross income which includes taxable income other than earnings (savings, dividends, etc.). To obtain the revenues required from the employer Y premium, the required rate would be about 0.67 percent under the basic-option benefits package and about 0.57 percent under the low-option package. To obtain the revenues required from the employee portion of the Y premium, the required rate would be about 0.65 percent under the basic-option plan and about 0.55 percent under the low-option plan.[22]

---

[22]The Y premium rate for individuals must be lower than the Y premium rate for employers, because the Y premium base for individuals is larger than the base for employers. If it is preferred to apply the same rate to both employers and individuals while meeting revenue requirements for benefits funded by the Y premium, the Y premium rate for both employers and employees would be set at 0.66 percent under the basic-option plan and 0.56 percent under the low-option plan.

As shown in Table 10, the effective X_1 fee base, which applies to employers who do not offer insurance, would be about $171 billion in 1988. The effective X_2 base, which applies to the amount of adjusted gross income above 150 percent of the poverty level up to the Social Security covered earnings amount ($45,000) for uninsured persons, would be about $206 billion. The X_2 base is larger than the X_1 base because: 1) the X_2 base includes incomes of both workers and non-workers while the X_1 base includes only workers, and 2) the X_2 base is based upon adjusted gross income which includes income other than earnings (savings, dividends, etc.). The fee rate necessary to generate the revenues required from the X_1 base would be about 9.68 percent under the basic-option plan and about 8.75 percent under the low-option plan. The rate required to generate the revenues required from the X_2 base would be about 2.04 percent under the basic-option plan and about 1.85 percent under the low-option plan.

Depending on the number of employers who elect to provide insurance rather than pay the fee, the amount of revenues obtained through the X_1 and X_2 fees may be smaller than shown in Table 10. However, the X_1 and X_2 rates required to fund the plan are likely to remain the same. This is because as employers elect to provide their own coverage, expenditures under the UNAC program will probably decline in proportion to the reduction in revenues.

However, the Y rates *will* change depending on the number of employers who elect to offer insurance. This is because the Y premium is intended to cover the cost of insuring workers and dependents below 150 percent of the poverty line. To the extent that employers offer coverage to workers below 150 percent of the poverty line, the revenues required from the Y premium will decline, resulting in lower Y premium rates.

Alternative Fee Bases

In its deliberations, the Commission considered alternative bases for the Y premium on employers and the X_2 fee on uninsured individuals. Estimates for the required rates are presented here.

1. Alternative Employer Y Premium Base. As discussed above, the Y health premium on employers would be a payroll fee calculated on wages and salaries for all workers up to the Social Security covered earnings level ($45,000 in 1988). One of the concerns the Commission had with this health premium base is that it would be applied uniformly across all firms regardless of the firms' financial position or profitability. Consequently, the Commission considered an employer Y premium on corporate **income** as an alternative to an employer premium based on

Table 9: Derivation of Effective Revenue Base for UNAC (in 1988 dollars)

Type of Fee	Fee Base Before Part-Time Worker Adjustment (in Billions)	Percent Included in Fee Base	Adjusted Fee Base (in Billions)	Part-Time Worker Adjustment (in Billions)	Effective Fee Base (in Billions)
Employer fees					
Y premium on wages and salaries for all workers up to $45,000[a]	$2,152.2	100.0%	$2,152.2	NA	$2,152.2
X$_1$ fee on payroll wages and salaries up to $45,000 for workers in plans that do not offer coverage	213.2	87.9	187.3	(15.8)	171.5
Self employed[b]	13.6	86.7	11.8	(1.0)	10.8
New businesses[c]					
Age one year	15.4	40.0	6.2	(0.5)	5.7
Age two years	14.9	60.0	8.9	(0.7)	8.2
Age three years	3.6	80.0	2.9	(0.2)	2.7
Small businesses (1–5 employees)[c]	40.9	80.0	32.7	(2.8)	29.9
Other employers	124.8	100.0	124.8	(10.6)	114.2
Individual fees					
Y premium on adjusted gross income above 150 percent of the poverty level up to $45,000[d]	2,206.4	100.0	2,206.4	NA	2,206.4
X$_2$ fee on adjusted gross income above 150 percent of the poverty line up to $45,000 for non-covered persons	226.9	99.2	225.0	(19.1)	205.9
Self employed[e]	14.5	86.7	12.6	(1.1)	11.5
Other persons	212.4	100.0	212.4	(18.0)	194.4

Source: Lewin/ICF estimates.

[a]The fee base estimate is based upon the Social Security Hospital Insurance Trust Fund Tax Base Estimates for 1988 provided by the actuaries of the Social Security Trust Funds. The base includes nearly all private sector and government employees.

[b]Based on Social Security Actuaries' estimates on total wages and salaries for self-employed persons covered by social security in 1988. It is estimated that about $14.7 billion of this income is attributed to uninsured persons who would be eligible to participate in the fund, based upon simulations using Health Benefits Simulation Model (HBSM). Due to credits provided self-employed persons under the social security, only about 80.6 percent of self-employment income is included in the effective tax base.

[c]Estimates based upon analysis of the Lewin/ICF Employer Health Benefits Survey database.

[d]Based on projections of adjusted gross income for 1988 adjusted to include only income above 150 percent of the poverty level and below $45,000.

[e]Includes self-employment income plus other taxable income up to $45,000. It is assumed that fee preferences for self-employed persons will be allowed such that 80.6 percent of this amount is included in the effective fee base.

Table 10: Fee Base Revenue Requirements and Requisite Fee Rates for UNAC (in 1988 dollars)[a]

Type of Fee	Effective Fee Base (in Billions)	Basic-option Plan		Low-option plan	
		Revenue Requirements (in Billions)	Requisite Fee Rate (Percent)	Revenue Requirements (in Billions)	Requisite Fee Rate (Percent)
Employer fees					
Y premium on wages and salaries for all workers up to $45,000	$2,152.2	14.4	0.67% (0.66)[b]	$12.2	0.57% (0.56)[b]
X_1 fee on payroll wages and salaries up to $45,000 for all workers in plans that do not offer coverage	171.5	16.6	9.68	15.0	8.75
Individual fees					
Y premiums on adjusted gross income above 150 percent of the poverty line up to $45,000	2,206.4	14.4	0.65 (0.66)[b]	12.2	0.55 (0.56)[b]
X_2 fee on adjusted gross income above 150 percent of the poverty line up to $45,000 for non-covered persons	205.9	4.2	2.04	3.8	1.85

Source: Lewin/ICF estimates using the Health Benefits Simulation Model (HBSM).
[a]All estimates include administrative costs.
[b]This is the fee rate if the Commission prefers to apply the same Y premium rate to both employers and individuals.

payroll. The intention was to concentrate the Y payment on the firms that can most afford the payment.

The simplest way to implement such a policy would be to establish the Y premium as a surcharge on federal corporate income taxes as determined under current law. In this alternative, the base is the amount of federal corporate income taxes paid which are estimated to be $99.0 billion in 1988. To raise the revenues required under the Y premium on employers under the basic-option benefits package ($14.4 billion in 1988), the Y surcharge rate would need to be set at 14.5 percent. Under the low-option benefits package the surcharge rate would need to be set at 12.3 percent.

Employers whose tax liabilities are small, which includes firms without net losses, will benefit substantially from establishing the Y premium as a surtax rather than a fee on payroll. It is important to note, however, that the Y premium on payroll will, on average, be less costly to the employer than will the surcharge even though both would raise the same amount of revenue. This is because the Y health premium can be deducted as a cost of doing business in determining net taxable corporate income just as Social Security is deductible under current law. Thus, the Y premium on payroll would be offset by a reduction in corporate tax payments while the surcharge, which is not deductible, would not be offset by corporate income tax savings.

2. Alternative X_2 Fee Base. Under the Commission's plan as currently proposed, the X_2 fee on uninsured individuals is applied to the amount of adjusted gross income above 150 percent of the poverty line up to the Social Security covered earnings level ($45,000 in 1988) for all uninsured persons. The Commission considered an alternative formulation of the X_2 fee, which would be based upon the **full** amount of adjusted gross income above 150 percent of the poverty level for uninsured persons. This would increase the X_2 fee base from $206 billion under the current plan to about $228 billion. Under the basic-option benefit package, this would reduce the X_2 rate from 2.04 percent under the current plan to about 1.84 percent. Under the low-option plan, the rate would decline from 1.85 percent under the current plan to about 1.67 percent. This change would also mean that wealthy uninsured individuals would pay quite a bit more in the X_2 fee than the actuarial amount of a comparable premium. Those individuals would likely purchase a private premium rather than pay the fee, reducing the X_2 base and thus, necessitating an increase in the X_2 rates.

Regional Fee Rate Variations

The Commission's proposal intends for the X fee rates to vary according to the variation in health care costs across states. Thus the X_1 and X_2 fee rates estimated here actually would vary by geographic region. In addition, states would be permitted, if they wished, to vary fee rates across regions within states, high- or low-wage occupational groups, and other factors related to the cost of medical care. Because health care costs vary across regions by as much as 20 percent, both across and within states, fee rates will vary widely across the nation.

This regional fee rate variation is intended to assure that the X_1 fee paid by individual employers reflects the level of health care costs in their geographic region. This will avoid creating a situation where nearly all firms in higher cost regions face substantial incentives to participate in the program rather than purchase insurance while only firms in lower cost regions have an incentive to purchase insurance rather than participate in the UNAC program.

The Y premium rates could be either uniform throughout the nation or varied by state. The advantage of setting nationwide Y premium rates is that revenues could be collected at the Federal level and allocated to states in proportion to need. This would permit cross-subsidization of program operations between upper and lower income states. The advantage of state-specific Y premium rates, however, is that states will have a greater incentive to implement cost control measures if they know that the savings will be reflected directly in the premiums charged within their state.

Fee Rates in Future Years

The various fee rates would be recalculated in each year to reflect the changing conditions facing the program. Each year, program administrators would redetermine the X and Y rates to reflect: 1) the growth in health care costs, 2) changes in the fee base (i.e., wage and salary levels), and 3) any revenue deficit/surplus under the program in the prior year. Many of the actuarial methods and operational guidelines used to set these rates could be patterned after those used by the actuaries of the Social Security Administration (SSA) in their annual redetermination of the Medicare Part B premium.[23]

The primary reason for recalibrating the various fee rates is that health care costs have been growing much faster than the wage bases to which the various fee rates are applied. For example, between 1983 and 1987, the health care component of the Consumer Price Index (CPI) grew at roughly two and one-half times the rate of growth in average weekly

---

[23]The actuaries of the SSA have developed procedures for projecting health expenditures which could be adapted for use by the program. The SSA actuaries have also developed guidelines for determining the appropriate level of reserve balances which also could be employed by the program.

earnings.[24] If this pattern continues (although it is predicted that cost control provisions in the Commission's plan could slow the rate of increase), expenditures under the program will grow relative to the various X and Y fee bases which will lead to higher X and Y fee rates over time.

The Commission's plan includes a provision intended to limit the increase in the X_1 fee rate over time. The plan would limit the X_1 fee rate such that the average employer X_1 fee payment (as a percentage of payroll) does not exceed 150 percent of the average commercial insurance premium cost in any particular state for the national basic benefits package (as a percentage of payroll) for firms that offer insurance. Any revenue shortfall created by this limitation on the X_1 fee rate would be covered by an increase in the Y rates. This provision is intended to limit health insurance costs as a percentage of payroll for firms participating in the program to within 150 percent of the level paid by other firms for the national basic benefits package required under the Commission's plan. This is intended to prevent the X_1 fee rate from increasing to such a high level that it substantially reduces employment among firms paying the X_1 fee.

The X and Y fee rates would also be set at levels which amortize any surplus or deficit experienced by the program in the prior year. For example, if the program experienced a deficit in the prior year, the X and Y fee rates for the next year would be set at a level which would both: 1) raise sufficient revenues to finance program expenditures projected for the next year, and 2) recover the prior year's deficit. Similarly, if the program experienced a surplus in the prior year, that surplus would be used to finance benefits in the following year which would offset any increase in the fee rates. This practice of amortizing year-to-year surpluses and deficits will assure that over the long term, expenditures and revenues under the fund will be in balance.

The potential for short-term deficits and surpluses suggests that the program should be equipped with the means to cope with fluctuations in fund balances. One approach would be to set the fee rates such that the program maintains a reserve balance which could be used to meet short-term revenue shortfalls. To deal with occasional deficits which exceed this reserve balance, the fund may also require some form of short-term borrowing authority.[25] These reserve balances and short-term borrowing capabilities will be important in dealing with cyclical economic patterns which may substantially increase program expenditures relative to the X and Y fee bases.

---

[24]"Economic Report of the President," February 1988.

[25]Such short-term borrowing could be accomplished through the sale of Treasury bonds arranged through the Federal Financing Bank (FFB).

Incentives and Impacts on Employers

Incentives Under UNAC[1]

The UNAC program is intended to provide coverage for a basic level of care for the uninsured and those currently under Medicaid. Therefore, the Commission plan offers incentives for employers to provide insurance, rather than allowing these people to go into the UNAC program— by requiring all employers who do not provide such coverage to pay a significant fee. In this section the incentives for employers to purchase insurance are explored. In addition, some options are discussed for **encouraging** employers to choose to provide insurance.

Firms that Now Provide Insurance

UNAC will affect existing employer plans in three major ways. First, many employers will be asked either to cover part-time workers who work over 25 hours a week or pay the X_1 fee on part-time employees. This could have an impact on firms that now offer insurance because most of these plans currently exclude part-time employees. A recent Lewin/ICF survey of employer health benefits indicates that about 65 percent of all uninsured part-time workers are employed by a firm which offers health benefits to full-time employees. Most employers will probably choose to pay the X_1 fee rather than purchase insurance because the X_1 fee payment on a part-time worker will on the average be about half the cost of purchasing insurance. This is because the X_1 fee, which is

---

[1]This section was taken largely from the analysis done for the Commission by Lewin/ICF.

calculated as a percentage of total earnings, will often be relatively small for part-time workers who typically have low earnings. Consequently, this analysis assumes that all employers choose to cover part-time workers under the program.

Several factors, however, will encourage employers to cover part-time workers rather than pay the X_1 fee. First, recent Internal Revenue Service (IRS) regulations, known as section 89 rules, will impose tax penalties on workers in firms which exclude significant portions of their work force from health insurance plans. The combined effect of these tax penalties and the X_1 fees may cause many employers to extend coverage to part-time workers. Second, employers seeking administrative simplicity may find it preferable to cover their entire work force rather than administer a separate fee system for part-time workers. Third, to the extent that coverage under the program is perceived to be inferior to standard employer coverage, many employers may be persuaded by employee sentiment to purchase coverage rather than pay the X_1 fee.

Second, some employers will have to pay the full amount of the X_1 fee unless they improve their plan benefits and premium sharing provisions to comply with minimum standards set by the Commission's proposal. Most employers who fall short of the minimum standards will probably choose to improve their plan rather than to pay the fee, however, because the cost of complying with the standards will nearly always be less than paying the full amount of the X_1 fee.

Lastly, some employers who currently offer health insurance will be eligible to participate in the program and will find it less costly to drop their health insurance plans and pay the fee. Most firms that currently offer insurance have average payrolls well above the level of 250 percent of the poverty threshold for an individual. However, it is estimated that about 1.9 million people are covered under an employer plan that falls below this average payroll standard. Under the Commission's plan, it will nearly always cost less for these firms to pay the X_1 fee than to purchase insurance. Consequently, it is likely that most of these firms will terminate their existing plans and pay the fee.[2]

Firms that Do Not Now Provide Insurance

We estimate that for firms with an average payroll per worker greater than 250 percent of the poverty threshold, very few would select cover-

---

[2]As discussed in Technical Appendix I, it is assumed that eligible firms terminate their existing plan to participate in the pool only if their plan also falls short of the minimum benefit and employer contribution standards set by the Commission's plan. Based on this assumption of the 1.9 million persons who could potentially be shifted to the pool, it is estimated that about 1.2 million will actually become covered under the pool.

age under UNAC. Many employers in tight labor markets may choose to purchase the insurance rather than pay the fee as a way of attracting desirable workers, although with universal health coverage, employer benefits might be less important in attracting workers. Under universal coverage, all persons are covered regardless of where or even if they work. In that situation, health benefits are likely to be an important factor in attracting desirable labor only to the extent that these benefits exceed the minimum levels of coverage mandated under the Commission's proposal. Employees may also prefer to be insured under an employer plan rather than a public health benefits system, which may carry with it some stigma.

On the other hand, due to the structure of the X_1 fee, employers face a substantial financial incentive to pay the fee rather than provide insurance. The X_1 fee rate is set at the level required to fund benefits only for workers and dependents above 150 percent of the poverty line. As discussed earlier, benefits under the program for workers and dependents below 150 percent of poverty are fully subsidized by revenues collected under the Y premium. Due to the Y premium subsidy, the cost of providing unsubsidized insurance would on average be about 50 percent greater than the X_1 fee payment.

The main explanation for the incentive to pay the X_1 fee rather than provide insurance is that most employers who do not offer insurance are small firms, and typically, premiums for small firms are higher than for larger groups because small groups present a larger potential risk relative to total premium payments than do large firms. Consequently, administrative overhead built into the premiums charged by small employers ranges between 12 and 25 percent of benefit payments. By comparison, we assume that the administrative overhead for benefits provided under the program will be about eight percent of benefit payments. Thus, the economies of scale realized by the program will, on average, lower the X_1 employer fee relative to the cost of purchasing insurance on the open market.

In some individual cases, employers may find that the cost of insuring workers will be less than the X_1 fee they would pay. The major reason for this is that insurance premiums vary based upon the characteristics of the groups being insured while the fee rate will be fixed across all demographic groups. A firm's X_1 fee payment will vary only with the earnings of the workers they employ. By contrast, the premium charged an employer will vary with the age, sex and family type (individual vs. family coverage) composition of the employer's work force. In addition, premiums often vary by 20 percent or more both across and within states due to regional variations in health care costs and treatment practices. Although the Commission's plan calls for X_1 fee variation by region and other factors, demographic variations across groups can still create variations in premiums relative to the X_1 fee. Consequently, firms facing high premiums generally will have an incentive to pay the fee while firms facing relatively low premiums will have an incentive to purchase the insurance.

Enhancing Incentives to Offer Coverage

The extreme variation in premium cost across groups makes it impractical to set an X_1 rate high enough to provide a universal incentive to purchase insurance. Raising the X_1 fee rate would also be contrary to the Commission's goal of keeping the X_1 fee low enough so that it does not discourage employment of lower wage workers. The primary reason that the X_1 fee is low relative to the cost of insurance is that the cost of covering workers and dependents below 150 percent of the poverty line is fully subsidized by the Y health premium. This subsidy reflects the Commission's principle that financing care for everyone, including the poor, is a shared responsibility. The X_1 fee rate cannot be set at a level which encourages employers to purchase insurance without compromising this important principle.

IMPACT ON EMPLOYERS

Nearly all employers will be affected by the Commission's plan. There are three ways in which the plan could affect employer costs. First, all employers who currently do not offer insurance will be required to offer a plan or pay the X_1 fee. Second, many employers who currently offer insurance will see increases in costs due to 1) the provision requiring coverage for part-time workers or X_1 fee payments and 2) the provisions setting standards for minimum benefits and minimum employer premium contributions. Third, increases in the cost of existing plans would be largely offset by reductions in costs due to the inter-employer equity provisions of the Commission's proposal. In this section, we describe the impact of the Commission's plan on employer costs.

Impact on Firms that Do Not Now Offer Coverage

Table 1 presents employer costs under the Commission's plan for firms that do not now offer coverage under the basic-option and low-option benefits packages by size of firm. For firms that do not now provide health benefits, the Commission's plan would result in an increase in employer costs of about $39 billion under the basic-option plan. As shown in Table 1, of this $39 billion increase in costs, about $23.6 billion would be attributed to employers that are expected to establish a health plan under the Commission's proposal (i.e., firms with an average payroll per employee above 250 percent of the poverty level), and about $15.4 billion would be X_1 fee payments by firms which participate in the program. Under the low-option plan, the total increase in costs for firms that do not now offer insurance would be about $35.4 billion of which about $21.4 billion would be attributed to firms required to establish a plan and about $14.0 billion would be X_1 fee payments by firms permitted to participate in the program.[3]

The estimates presented in Table 1 assume that all firms eligible to participate in the program will choose to do so. The cost to employers would be quite different if these employers choose instead to purchase insurance for their employees. Table 2 compares costs for firms which participate in the program under two alternative scenarios: 1) all eligible employers choose to pay the X_1 fee, and 2) all firms elect to offer coverage to uninsured workers. These estimates indicate that, on average, paying the X_1 fee will be substantially less costly to the employer than providing insurance. As shown in Table 2, under the basic-option benefits package, total costs to employers would be about $23 billion if all eligible employers purchase insurance, whereas employer costs would be only about $15.4 billion if all of these employers elect to pay the X_1 fee.

The X_1 fee tends to be the least costly alternative for eligible firms for two reasons. First, the X_1 fee rate is set at the level required to finance benefits for workers and dependents with incomes above 150 percent of the poverty line. Coverage for workers and dependents below 150 percent of the poverty line is fully subsidized by the Y premium. Due to this substantial Y premium subsidy, the X_1 fee payment will on average be significantly less than the cost of commercial insurance, the cost of which is completely unsubsidized.

Second, it is likely that the program can provide the benefits at a lower cost than can private insurers. One reason for this is that most firms that do not offer insurance are small employers who typically pay a much higher premium than do larger employers. The premium for small groups is usually higher than for large groups because private insurers generally include in small group premiums a higher administrative surcharge ranging from 12 to 25 percent of benefit payments to cover the

---

[3]The employer cost estimates for firms establishing a plan include the employer share of the premium, which is assumed to be 75 percent of total premium costs, and the X_1 fee payment by these firms for part-time workers.

Table 1: Impact of UNAC on Employer Costs for Firms that Do Not Now Offer Insurance (in billions)

Firm Size	Basic-option Benefits Package			Low-option Benefits Package		
	All Firms	Firms that Establish Health Plans[a]	Firms that Pay the X_1 Fee[b]	All Firms	Firms that Establish Health Plans[a]	Firms that Pay the X_1 Fee
Under 25 employees	$12.6	$8.4	$4.2	$11.4	$7.6	$3.8
25–99 employees	5.6	3.4	2.2	5.1	3.1	2.0
100–499 employees	5.4	3.0	2.4	4.9	2.7	2.2
500 or more employees	15.4	8.8	6.6	14.0	8.0	6.0
All firms	$39.0	$23.6	$15.4	$35.4	$21.4	$14.0

Source: Lewin/ICF estimates.

[a]Employer costs for firms the Commission expects will purchase insurance rather than pay the X_1 fee. These include all firms that do not now offer insurance who have an average payroll per employee above 250 percent of the poverty level ($14,000 in 1988). Costs include administrative charges anticipated in the open market ranging from an average of 17 percent in small firms to 6.5 percent in large firms. Excludes employee share of premium contribution (25 percent). Includes X_1 fee payments for part-time workers of $2.0 billion under the basic-option plan and $1.8 billion under the low-option plan.

[b]These include all employers who have an average annual payroll per worker which is less than 250 percent of the poverty level.

Table 2: Distribution of UNAC Costs for Firms Who Participate in the UNAC Programs Under Alternative Scenarios in 1988[a] (in billions)

Firm Size	Basic-option Benefits Package		Low-option Benefits Package	
	Scenario 1: All Firms Pay the X_1 Fee[b]	Scenario 2: All Firms Purchase Insurance[c]	Scenario 1: All Firms Pay the X_1 Fee[b]	Scenario 2: All Firms Purchase Insurance[c]
Under 25 employees	$4.2	$9.2	$3.8	$8.3
25–99 employees	2.2	2.8	2.0	2.5
100–499 employees	2.4	2.6	2.2	2.4
500 or more employees	6.6	8.4	6.0	7.6
All firms	$15.4	$23.0	$14.0	$20.8

Source: Lewin/ICF estimates.

[a] Firms participating in the UNAC program which have an average payroll per employee below 250 percent of the poverty threshold for a single individual ($14,000 in 1988).

[b] Assumes all firms pay the X_1 fee rather than provide insurance.

[c] Employer costs assuming all eligible firms choose to purchase insurance rather than pay the X_1 fee. Includes administrative charges anticipated in the open market ranging from an average of 17 percent in small firms to 6.5 percent in large firms. Excludes employee share of premium contribution (25 percent). Includes X_1 fee payments for part-time workers.

greater risk associated with insuring a small group.[4] By comparison, we assume that the administrative charges under the program will be about 8 percent of benefit payments. Because this lower administrative charge is included in the calculation of the X_1 fee rate, the X_1 fee payment tends to be lower than the employer cost of providing insurance.

The program also will be able to take advantage of certain economies of scale which may not be achievable by commercial insurers. For example, it is likely that the program, which will cover about 68 million persons, will be able to negotiate more advantageous reimbursement rates with providers than will smaller insurers. To the extent this occurs, this will further reduce the X_1 fee relative to the cost of insurance.[5]

Impact on Employers that Now Offer Insurance

The Commission's proposal would have a significant impact on many employers who now offer health insurance coverage. To avoid paying the X_1 fee, the Commission's plan requires that employers offer a minimum standard package of benefits and limit the employee contribution for these benefits to 25 percent of the total premium (the employee may pay a greater percentage of the costs for benefits above the minimum benefit standard). If the employer does not comply with these provisions, the employer will pay the full amount of the X_1 fee for all employees. Also, the employer must either cover part-time workers or pay the X_1 fee for part-time workers.

The Commission's plan also includes provisions that will benefit employers who currently provide insurance. First, as discussed above, the plan 1) expects that working dependents take coverage through their own job or with a wraparound from their spouse's employer, or that they pay the X_2 fee, and 2) assigns responsibility for insuring dependent children by having one parent pick up the children in cases where both parents work. These provisions will shift the cost of insuring some working dependent spouses and some dependent children away from employers who now offer coverage to employers who do not now cover their workers. Second, by providing coverage to the uninsured, the

---

[4]Small groups present a greater loss risk relative to total premium payments than do larger groups. For example, in some small groups a single catastrophic illness may cost more than total group premium payments. This risk factor accounts for the large administrative overhead charges assessed on groups. The data on the typical administrative surcharge for small groups are based upon Lewin/ICF consultation with health benefit actuaries.

[5]The potential savings resulting from these economies of scale were not estimated in this study and are not reflected in our estimates of pool benefit payments.

Commission's plan would greatly reduce charity care by providers which will result in substantial savings to employers who currently offer insurance. This is because provider charges typically include an overhead charge for the cost of providing uncompensated care. This overhead charge would be drastically reduced by this plan due to the reduction in charity care (it is likely that some charity care will continue for the homeless and for aliens).

As shown in Table 3, total health plan premiums for employers who currently offer insurance would be about $123.1 billion in 1988 of which about $99.3 billion would be financed by employer premium payments and about $23.8 billion would be financed by employee premium contributions. Under the basic-option plan, the Commission's proposal limiting employee contributions to 25 percent of total premiums would reduce the employee share of premium payments by about $6.1 billion, all of which now would be paid by employers. Under the low-option plan, employer premium contributions would increase by about $5.7 billion.

The requirement that plans provide a minimum standard package of benefits would increase employer costs by about $3.2 billion under the basic-option benefit package. Under the low-option package benefit improvements will increase costs in existing plans by about $2.9 billion. We assume that the level of benefits provided by plans which are currently more generous than the minimum benefit standard will be retained. This is because many of the most generous plans are established through collective bargaining agreements that are likely to be retained.[6]

As discussed above, we assume that all employers that do not now offer insurance to part-time workers will choose to cover these workers under the program by paying the X_1 fee rather than by providing insurance. As shown in Table 3, under the basic-option plan, we estimate that the cost of insuring part-time workers under the fund will be about $3.5 billion, about $2.8 billion of which would be X_1 fee payments by employers and about $0.7 billion would be X_2 fee payments by workers. Under the low-option plan, the cost of insuring part-time workers would be about $3.2 billion of which $2.6 billion would be X_1 fee payments by employers and $0.6 billion would be employee X_2 fee payments. How-

---

[6]As we discussed above, we assume that employers who currently offer insurance will transfer their employees to the pool if 1) they have an average payroll per worker below 250 percent of poverty and 2) they are in a plan which falls short of the minimum benefit and employer contribution standards. Using these assumptions, we estimate that about 1.2 million people covered by existing plans will be transferred to the pool and their employees will now pay the X_1 fee. The resulting change in costs for employers who now provide insurance is included in Table 3 in the estimates of the cost of complying with the minimum benefit and employer contribution standards.

Table 3: Impact of UNAC on Employers Who Currently Offer Coverage (amounts in billions of 1988 dollars)[a]

	Basic-option Plan			Low-option Plan		
	Employer Plan Costs*	Employer Share†	Employee Share‡	Employer Plan Costs*	Employer Share†	Employee Share‡
Current law in 1988	$123.1	$99.3	$23.8	$123.1	$99.3	$23.8
Change in plan costs under policy by provision						
Impact of minimum benefit standard						
Plan premium improvements[b]	NA	6.1	(6.1)	NA	5.7	(5.7)
Improvement in plan provisions[c]	3.2	3.2	NA	2.9	2.9	NA
Cost of insuring part-time workers[d]	3.5	2.8	0.7	3.2	2.6	0.6
Dependents who become covered on plan[e]	1.5	1.3	0.2	1.5	1.3	0.2
Working dependents who become covered on their own job[f]	(17.2)	(14.7)	(2.5)	(17.2)	(14.7)	(2.5)
Children allocated to other plans[g]	(4.7)	(4.1)	(0.6)	(4.7)	(4.1)	(0.6)
Premium reduction attributed to elimination of charity care overhead charges by providers	(4.9)	(4.2)	(0.7)	(4.4)	(3.8)	(0.6)
Total plan costs under Commission plan in 1988	$104.5	$89.7	$14.8	$104.4	$89.2	$15.2

Source: Lewin/ICF estimates using the Household Benefit Simulation Model (HBSM).

NA = Not applicable.

[a] All plan premium cost estimates presented in this table include a surcharge of 8 percent for administration. Components may not sum to totals due to rounding.

[b] The plan requires that employees contribute no more than 25 percent of the premium for a minimum standard package of benefits. The employee is permitted to pay a greater share of the premium for benefits above the standard.

[c] Employers are required to provide a minimum standard package of benefits.

[d] We assume that all employers who do not now cover part-time workers will elect to pay the X_1 fee for part-time employees to cover them under the UNAC program. The employer share of the cost shown here is the X_1 fee payment while the employee share is the amount of the X_2 fee payment.

[e] We assume that all covered workers with dependents who have not elected the family coverage option will elect family coverage rather than pay the X_2 fee.

[f] Existing employer plans would no longer provide coverage to working dependents. Working dependents will be required to take coverage on their own employer's plan or pay the X_2 fee and become covered under the Commission's plan.

[g] In the case of families with two working parents, responsibility for insuring dependent children will be allocated across the parents' employer plans.

[*] Includes total plan premium.

[†] Premium paid by the employer.

[‡] Includes the portion of the plan premium paid by the employee.

ever, if employers choose to insure part-time workers under their own plan rather than pay the X_1 fee, employer plan costs would be about $7.8 billion, of which about $6.7 billion would be paid by employers and about $1.1 billion would be paid by employees in the form of premium contributions.

We also estimate that under current policy there are about 1.6 million dependents of covered workers who are not covered because the worker chooses not to elect the family coverage option. We assume that workers would elect to cover these dependents to avoid paying the X_2 fee. As shown in Table 3, we estimate that this would increase costs for employers who now offer insurance by about $1.3 billion.

As shown in Table 3, the Commission expects that working dependents obtain coverage through their own employment which would reduce costs for existing employer plans by about $17.2 billion. The plan calls for children to be covered under one parent's plan when two parents work, reducing costs in existing plans by about $4.7 billion. Together, these inter-employer equity provisions would reduce the employer share of premium payments by about $18.8 billion and reduce the employee share of premium payments by about $3.1 billion (we assume that savings in plan costs will be reflected in both the employer and the employee premium payment). These savings could be smaller, however, if employers elect to offer coverage to working dependent spouses (as discussed above, employers have the option of offering wraparound coverage to working spouses). Also, because charity care overhead charges by providers are reduced under this proposal, employer plan costs would be reduced by about $4.9 billion under the basic-option plan and $4.4 billion under the low-option plan.

The net impact of these provisions would be to reduce total health plan[7] costs for both employers and employees in existing plans. As shown in Table 3, total employer premium payments would decline from about $99.3 billion under current policy to about $89.7 billion under the basic-option plan and about $89.2 billion under the low-option plan. Total employee premium contributions for existing plans would decline from about $23.8 billion to about $14.8 billion under the basic-option plan and about $15.2 billion under the low-option plan.

---

[7]As discussed above, the total amount of charity care which would become covered by the pool would be about $5.7 billion under the basic-option plan and about $5.3 billion under the low-option plan. It was assumed that these charity care savings will be distributed across group and non-group plans. Under this assumption, the portion of these savings attributed to current employers will be $4.9 billion under the basic-option plan and $4.4 billion under the low-option plan. This also assumes that providers pass on the full amount of charity care savings to health care consumers in the form of slowed growth in health care charges.

Total After-Tax Employer Costs

The total after-tax cost to employers under this proposal would be the total increase in employer costs less any reduction in corporate income tax payments arising from the deductibility of employee benefit expenses.[8] In this study, the before-tax cost to the employer under this proposal is the net increase in employer premium payments, plus the amount of the employer X_1 and Y premium payments. The after-tax employer cost is the before-tax cost less any reduction in corporate income taxes resulting from these increased employer expenses.

For firms that now offer health coverage to some or all of their employees, we estimate that the after-tax net change in employer costs would be an increase of about $1.4 billion under the basic-option plan and a reduction of about $100 million under the low-option plan. As shown in Table 4 for firms that currently offer insurance, the total before-tax costs under the Commission's proposal would be about $2 billion under the basic-option benefits package. This includes employer Y premium payments of about $11.6 billion and X_1 fee payments for part-time workers of $2.8 billion less net savings in health benefit payments of about $12.4 billion (as explained in the prior section, employers who currently offer insurance would see a net reduction in health benefit payments primarily due to the inter-employer equity provisions of the Commission's proposal). Because this net increase in employer costs of $2 billion is deductible under the corporate income tax, this increase in costs would be offset by a reduction in corporate income tax payments of about $600 million.

The after-tax net increase in costs for firms that do not now offer insurance would be about $25.9 billion under the basic-option plan and about $23.4 billion under the low-option plan. As shown in Table 4, for firms that currently do not offer a health plan to any of their employees, the before-tax cost to employers would be about $38.2 billion under the basic-option benefits package. As shown in Table 4, this includes the Y premium payment of about $2.8 billion, the X_1 fee payment of about $13.8 billion for employees covered under the fund, and expenditures of $21.6 billion for persons covered under newly established plans. These increases in employer costs would be offset by a reduction in corporate income taxes of about $12.3 billion.

These estimates indicate that the Commission's plan will have a significant impact on Federal corporate income tax revenues. As shown

---

[8]These corporate income tax savings arise from the fact that employers are permitted to deduct employee health benefit payments and payroll tax payments such as X_1 and Y premiums, as a cost of doing business in determining net taxable income.

Table 4: Change in Employer Costs Under UNAC (in billions)

Plan Provisions[c]	All Firms		Firms that Currently Offer Insurance[a]		Firms that Currently Do Not Offer Insurance[b]	
	Basic-option Benefits Package	Low-option Benefits Package	Basic-option Benefits Package	Low-option Benefits Package	Basic-option Benefits Package	Low-option Benefits Package
Coverage mandate[c]	$21.6	$19.6	NA	NA	$21.6	$19.6
Minimum standards provisions[d]	(12.4)	(12.7)	(12.4)	(12.7)	NA	NA
X_1 fee payments[e]	16.6	15.0	2.8	2.6	13.8	12.4
Y premium[f]	14.4	12.2	11.6	9.9	2.8	2.3
Net change in employer costs before taxes	40.2	34.1	2.0	(0.2)	38.2	34.3
Corporate income tax offset[g]	(12.9)	(10.8)	(0.6)	0.1	(12.3)	(10.9)
After tax net cost to employers	$27.3	$23.3	$1.4	($0.1)	$25.9	$23.4

Source: Lewin/ICF estimates.

NA = Not applicable.

[a]Includes all firms that currently offer insurance regardless of whether or not part-time workers are excluded.

[b]Includes all firms that do not offer insurance to any of their employees.

[c]Includes firms required to provide insurance to workers.

[d]Includes the minimum actuarial standard, the maximum employee contribution standard, charity care savings, and the redistribution of benefit payments across employers resulting from the inter-employer equity provisions. Also includes change in employer costs resulting from transfer of individuals to the program.

[e]We assume that all employers who currently do not offer insurance and have employers averaging less than 250 percent of the poverty level choose to pay the X_1 fee rather than provide insurance. For firms that currently offer insurance, this includes X_1 fee payments for part-time workers and firms which transfer coverage to the program.

[f]Includes only employer Y premium payments.

[g]Assumes an average corporate income tax rate of 32 percent. Also assumes that X_1 fees and Y premium are deductible as are payroll taxes.

in Table 4, Federal corporate tax revenues would be reduced by about $12.9 billion under the basic-option plan and about $10.8 billion under the low-option plan.

Impact on Employment and Wage Levels

Employers could respond to the increase in costs by either increasing prices for the goods and services they produce or by reducing other forms of employee compensation. The general consensus among economists, however, is that, in the long run, few employers would respond by raising prices. This is largely because many of the firms affected by this proposal are small firms, many of whom are in the service and retail trade industries, that typically have little control over the prices they can charge in their markets. It is more likely that the increase in employer costs under the Commission's plan will result in some changes in levels of employment and/or wage rates.

Most economists believe that employers will respond to the increase in costs resulting from health insurance mandates and/or fee incentives by reducing wage levels and other forms of employee compensation (e.g., pensions and life insurance) rather than reducing their work force. This judgment is based largely upon the economic theory that, in the long run, wage levels adjust so that employee compensation costs, which include health insurance premiums and payroll-related taxes and fees such as the X_1 and Y premiums, conform to the marginal product of the work force.

However, the Commission's plan could result in some loss of jobs for those employed at or near the minimum wage ($3.35 per hour in most states). This is because the minimum wage law prohibits employers from adjusting wages below this level. Due to this rigidity in wage levels for minimum wage workers, it is possible that there would be a loss of employment among workers who are at or near the minimum wage. The Congressional Budget Office (CBO) estimates that under an employer-mandated plan there may be a reduction in minimum wage employment of about 100,000 jobs.[9]

The number of jobs lost under the Commission's plan, however, is likely to be less than under a simple employer-mandated plan. This is because 1) due to Y premium subsidies of coverage for low wage workers, the X_1 fee is significantly less than the cost of commercial insurance, and 2) for part-time workers, the Commission's plan scales downward the X_1 fee rate in proportion to the number of hours worked which tends

---

[9]See: CBO Testimony on S.1265/H.R. 2508.

to lessen the impact of the Commission's plan on minimum wage workers, many of whom are employed only part time.

Any reduction in employment occurring as a result of the Commission's plan will be offset in part by an increase in employment in the health care industry as the availability of health insurance leads to increases in the utilization of health care services. However, it is unlikely that a significant portion of these new jobs will be filled by displaced minimum wage workers. Instead, most of the increase in employment will be for nurses and other skilled professionals rather than for entry-level workers.

While in the long run we anticipate only a relatively small reduction in employment levels, the short-run impacts of the Commission's plan could be substantial. This is because 1) many employee compensation packages are determined through collective bargaining agreements which cannot be altered in the short run, and 2) even in the absence of collective bargaining agreements, it is often impractical for employers to impose abrupt pay cuts and benefit reductions on their employees. These short-run rigidities in employee compensation could result in hardships for some employers and some short-term loss of jobs. One way to lessen these short-run impacts is to phase in the Commission's plan over a number of years so that employers can plan on these cost increases when setting employee compensation levels.

Potential Savings Generated by the Implementation of Practice Guidelines[1]

Recent research findings have raised serious questions about the appropriateness of many health care interventions. These findings suggest that many medical practices are not rigorously tested; in fact, procedures often proliferate despite the absence of adequate knowledge about their appropriateness, clinical effectiveness or potential outcomes. There is increasing evidence that health professionals do not have adequate access to information about the risks, benefits, and outcomes of alternative medical practices. Researchers have suggested there is a need for better information on the relative effectiveness of alternative interventions and for the development of practice guidelines that would inform clinical decisionmaking.

The National Leadership Commission suggests that the combined Federal/private investment in developing guidelines and advancing health services research should be increased over five years to an annual rate of $500 million.

This section estimates the potential cost-savings that could be generated by the widespread adoption of practice guidelines in the medical care system. It provides an estimate of potential savings and discusses the rationale and methods. Clearly, any savings generated by the widespread adoption of practice guidelines would be offset to some extent by the investment in research; these estimates do not account for the offset.

---

[1]Adapted from a Commission-sponsored Lewin/ICF analysis.

Nor do they include the cost of improvements in substandard care that might result from the implementation of guidelines or the cost of adopting and enforcing guidelines.

Two separate approaches were employed to discuss how much savings might result from the adoption of clinical practice guidelines. In the first approach, the possible effects of changes in practice patterns on the growth of health care service intensity in the future were considered. In the second approach, the potential for reducing costs through eliminating inappropriate services in the present level of care being provided was considered. The findings are outlined here, while the methods are described in Appendix F.

SAVINGS DUE TO REDUCTIONS IN FUTURE INTENSITY GROWTH

Estimates of future intensity growth are really a calculated residual that embrace a wide range of changes, over time, in the mix of inputs used by health care practitioners. As such, "intensity" is driven as much by changes in patient preferences as by conscious changes in the way that physicians practice medicine.

To compute the intensity residual, official projections of growth in health care expenditures over the 1989–1993 period were "deflated" with adjustments for input price changes and population growth. To provide a range of potential values, estimates for the Medicare program (using OMB estimates of five-year program costs), and for the national health expenditures as a whole (using estimates from the National Health Expenditures accounts), were calculated separately.

Medicare

The amount of projected cost growth due to rising intensity of service in the Medicare program for Part A and Part B were calculated separately. Table 1 presents the estimated Medicare budget for Part A, and estimates of the portion of this budget that is attributable to service intensity.

A similar set of estimates is presented for Part B of the Medicare program in Table 2. The amount of the budget attributable to intensity equals approximately $3 billion for Part B in FY 90.

Total Population

Table 3 presents similar estimates relating to all health expenditures. It suggests that for hospital expenditures, as much as $72 billion is attributable to service intensity in estimated 1993 spending.

Table 1: Part A Budget and Portion of the Budget Attributable to Service Intensity: FY 89–FY 93 (in billions)

	FY 89	FY 90	FY 91	FY 92	FY 93
Part A budget	$57.0	$63.6	$70.0	$76.6	$83.2
Portion attributable to service intensity*	NA	$4.1–4.7	$8.7–9.8	$13.6–15.2	$18.4–20.9

Source: Office of Management and Budget.
*Range is provided because different inflation projections yielded different estimates.

Table 2: Part B Budget and Portion of Part B Budget Attributable to Service Intensity: FY 89–FY 93 (in billions)

	FY 89	FY 90	FY 91	FY 92	FY 93
Part B budget	$39.7	$44.9	$51.1	$58.4	$66.5
Portion attributable to service intensity*	NA	$2.9–3.6	$6.3–7.8	$9.9–12.7	$13.9–18.2

Source: Office of Management and Budget.
*Range is provided because different inflation projections yielded different estimates.

Table 3: National Health Expenditures for Hospital and Physicians Services: Estimated Budgets and Portion of Budget Attributable to Service Intensity: FY 89–FY 93 (in billions)

	FY 89	FY 90	FY 91	FY 92	FY 93
Hospital					
Total budget	$228.5	250.4	$274.9	$300.9	$329.1
Attributed to intensity*	NA	$13.5–15.8	$28.9–33.3	$45.6–52.1	$62.5–72.7
Physician					
Total budget	$120.9	$132.6	$145.8	$160.3	$175.2
Attributed to intensity*	NA	$7.2–9.1	$14.9–19.3	$22.9–30.9	$31.2–42.9

Source: Health Care Financing Administration, Office of the Actuary.
*Range is provided because different inflation projections yielded different estimates.

What Can Be Saved from Changes in Practice Patterns

The effect of changes in practice patterns on the growth of service intensity is difficult to estimate with precision. Some amount of increased service intensity is undoubtedly due to appropriate changes in medical practice—changes that would be validated by whatever guidelines were applied. Thus, it is neither expected nor desirable that the entire amount attributable to service intensity be "saved." Nevertheless, the estimates presented in Tables 1–3 represent the portion of the budget that could be potentially affected by changes in practice.

The Health Care Financing Administration (HCFA) and the Prospective Payment Assessment Commission (ProPAC) have in the past considered this issue as part of their efforts to determine the appropriate factor to update for Medicare's prospective payment system (PPS). HCFA has estimated that as much as two percentage points of the annual hospital intensity index would be influenced by practice pattern changes, notably through reductions in average length of stay.[2]

If this rule were generalized to include both physician and hospital services, it would imply that potential "savings" of two percentage points of the currently projected growth rate could be influenced by changes in practice patterns. Tables 4 and 5 present those estimates of potential savings. Over a four-year period, this amounts to a policy target of about $5.9 billion annually for Medicare Parts A and B combined. For national health expenditures, the total policy target for fiscal years 90 through 93 is $84 billion, or an average of $22 billion annually.

SAVINGS DUE TO THE ELIMINATION OF UNNECESSARY PROCEDURES

As a second method of approximating the potential effects of changing practice patterns on health care costs, a "bottom up" estimate of the potential for savings through reducing the volume of inappropriate ser-

Table 4: National Health Expenditures for Hospital and Physician Services: Estimate of Cumulative Savings Due to Reductions in Future Intensity Growth (in billions)

	FY 89	FY 90	FY 91	FY 92	FY 93
Hospital	$228.5	$250.4	$274.9	$300.9	$329.1
Physician	120.9	132.6	145.8	160.3	175.2
Total	349.4	383.0	420.7	461.2	504.3
Total budget at approximately 2 percentage points less		375.9	405.3	436.1	467.9
Savings*		7.1	15.4	25.1	36.4

*Estimated savings, years 2–5: $84 billion.

―――――――

[2]Federal Register, 1985.

Table 5: Medicare Expenditures for Hospital and Physician Services: Estimate of Cumulative Savings Due to Reduction in Future Intensity Growth (in billions)

	FY 89	FY 90	FY 91	FY 92	FY 93
Part A	$57.0	$63.6	$70.0	$76.6	$83.2
Part B	39.7	44.9	51.1	58.4	66.5
Total	96.7	108.5	121.1	135.0	149.7
Total budget at approximately 2 percentage points less		106.6	116.8	127.9	139.3
Savings*		1.9	4.3	7.1	10.4

*Estimated savings, years 2–5: $23.73 billion.

vices now being provided was developed. There is, at present, no comprehensive accounting of inappropriate services; research is just beginning to provide evidence permitting quantification of such service volume.

Accordingly, this methodology is directed at an estimate of potential savings in a short list of selected procedures that have been the focus of early research in this area. It is expected that the ultimate payoff from more in-depth research on a wider range of procedures would yield savings **significantly larger** than the amount estimated for the nine procedures selected in this analysis.

Medicare

Using Medicare Part B claims, it was estimated that a total of approximately $1.4 billion was paid by the carriers to physicians for the nine procedures listed in Table 6. This list represents high-volume, high-cost procedures for which many believe practice guidelines are warranted. For procedures for which estimates were available (largely from the RAND Corporation), costs that potentially would be avoided due to the elimination of their inappropriate use were calculated.

When considering procedures for which estimates were not available, it was assumed that approximately 5 percent of total volume might be eliminated by the application of guidelines. These calculations suggest that, for the nine procedures selected, eliminating the indicated volumes of services would reduce costs by approximately $150.7 million for the Part B program alone. Additional savings would be generated by the elimination of procedures not included on this list. In addition, savings would accrue for the Part A program if the elimination of these

Table 6: Potential Part B Savings Attributable to the Elimination of Unnecessary or Inappropriate Care for Nine Selected Procedures (in millions)

Procedure	Total Part B Allowed Charges (1987)	Estimated Rate of Inappropriate Use	Estimated Savings by Procedure
Hip replacement	$154.6	5.0%[1]	$7.7
Knee replacement	99.0	5.0	4.9
Pacemaker insertion	73.6	17.0[2]	12.5
Coronary artery bypass graft (CABG)	279.3	14.0[3]	39.1
Carotid endarterectomy	93.9	32.4[3]	30.4
Upper GI endoscopy	177.8	17.2[3]	30.6
Colonoscopy	240.6	5.0	12.0
Transurethral resection of the prostate	235.5	5.0	11.8
Hysterectomy	34.8	5.0	1.7
Totals	$1,389.1		$150.7

[1]We assumed that 5 percent of procedures might be eliminated for procedures for which we do not have data.

[2]Source: Greenspan et al., 1988.

[3]Source: Respectively, Winslow et al., 1988a; Winslow et al., 1988b; Kahn et al., 1988.

procedures were also to result in averting a hospitalization that would otherwise have occurred.

Total Population

A second set of calculations was performed to estimate potential costs averted due to the elimination of unnecessary or inappropriate care population-wide. We believe that eliminating 5 percent of the number of all the high-volume, high-cost procedures listed in Table 7 would save as much as $1.3 billion in FY 90. We selected a 5 percent figure as a conservative estimate, representing the minimum that might be saved. Assuming a 4 percent growth rate in health expenditures annually, this estimate could near $1.5 billion by FY 93.

DISCUSSION

These analyses suggest that elimination of inappropriate or unnecessary care would generate savings far in excess of the investment required;

Table 7: Potential Savings to the Health System Resulting from Reducing the Volume of Eleven Selected Procedures by Five Percent (in millions)

Procedure	Total Dollar Savings Per Procedure
Hip replacement	$66.9
Total knee replacement	100.7
Pacemaker insertion	73.5
Coronary artery bypass graft (CABG)	245.1
Carotid endarterectomy	51.7
Upper GI endoscopy	8.4
Cholecystectomy	339.4
Transurethral resection of the prostate	65.6
Hysterectomy	195.9
Cesarean section	160.2
Totals	$1,307.4

however, some caveats regarding the interpretation of these data apply. For example, the estimates provided:

- Do not account for the cost of "administering" practice guidelines.

- Fail to account for improvements in the quality of care, or in access to care that might result from the adoption of guidelines.

- Fail to account for the potential cost of alternative treatments that might be substituted for procedures determined to be inappropriate.

- Represent a mix of data from a variety of sources (discussed in Appendix A) and thus the data should be viewed solely as "ballpark figures."

- Fail to account for the fact that programs designed to eliminate inappropriate care could never be 100 percent effective.

SELECTED BIBLIOGRAPHY

"The Cesarean Future," *Medical Benefits*, October 31, 1987.

Federal Register, Health Care Financing Administration, "Medicare Program: Changes to the Inpatient Prospective Payment System and Fiscal Year 1986 Rates; Proposed Rules," June 10, 1985, pp. 24366–24497.

Greenspan, A., Kay, H., et al., "Incidence of Unwarranted Implantation of Permanent Cardiac Pacemakers in a Large Medical Population," *NEJM* 318(3):158–163, January 21, 1988.

Kahn, K., Kosecoff, J., et al., "The Use and Misuse of Upper Gastrointestinal Endoscopy," *Annals of Internal Medicine* 109:664–670, 1988.

U.S. Department of Health and Human Services, National Center for Health Statistics, *Detailed Diagnoses and Procedures for Patients Discharged from Short-stay Hospitals, United States, 1985*, Series 13(90), Publication 87–1751, April 1987.

"Results of Second Opinion Program for Coronary Artery Bypass Graft Surgery," *Medical Benefits*, October 31, 1987.

Winslow, C., Kosecoff, J., et al., "The Appropriateness of Performing Coronary Artery Bypass Surgery," *JAMA* 260(4):505–509, July 22/29, 1988.

Winslow, C., Solomon, D., et al., "The Appropriateness of Carotid Endarterectomy," *NEJM* 318(12):721–727, March 24, 1988.

⌐┘ └⌐
Appendix A
⌐┐ ┌⌐

Commission and Adviser Biographies

COMMISSION MEMBERS

Co-chairmen

Robert D. Ray, J.D., is Co-chairman of the National Leadership Commission on Health Care and President and Chief Executive Officer of Blue Cross and Blue Shield of Iowa. He is the former President of Life Investors Insurance Company of America. From 1969 to 1983, Mr. Ray served as Governor of Iowa. In 1975-76 he was Chairman of the National Governors' Association. Prior to 1969, Mr. Ray was a partner in the law firm of Lawyer, Lawyer and Ray. Mr. Ray is the recipient of eleven honorary degrees, and currently sits on the Boards of Directors of several corporations, including I.E. Industries and the Maytag Company. He is also a trustee of Drake University, the Iowa Natural Heritage Foundation and the Herbert Hoover Foundation. Mr. Ray received a B.A. degree in Business from Drake University in 1952 and a J.D. degree in 1954, also from Drake.

Paul G. Rogers, LL.B., is Co-chairman of the National Leadership Commission on Health Care and an attorney with Hogan & Hartson in Washington, D.C. Mr. Rogers was a member of Congress representing Florida from 1955 to 1979 and served as Chairman of the Subcommittee on Health and the Environment of the Committee on Energy and Commerce from 1971 to 1979. As a Congressman, Mr. Rogers played a major role in enacting numerous pieces of health-related legislation such as: The National Cancer Act; the Health Manpower Training Act; the Heart, Blood Vessel, Lung and Blood Act; The Research on Aging Act of 1970; the Medical Devices Amendments of 1976; the Emergency Medical Services Act; the Health Maintenance Organization Act; the Clear Air Act; the Safe Drinking Water Act; and the Radiation Health Safety Act. Mr. Rogers graduated from the University of Florida Law School after serving with the Army for four years in Europe.

President

Henry E. Simmons, M.D., M.P.H., F.A.C.P., is President of the National Leadership Commission on Health Care and a visiting Research Professor of Health Services Administration at the School of Government and Business, The George Washington University. Prior to the Commission's formation, Dr. Simmons was Vice President and Director, Health Care Division, Sears World Trade, Inc. from 1983 to 1985. Dr. Simmons also has five years of federal service as Director, Bureau of Drugs, of the Food and Drug Administration; Deputy Assistant Secretary for Health; and Director of the Office of Professional Standards Review, all within the Department of Health, Education and Welfare. Dr. Simmons was full-time Faculty and Consultant in Rheumatic Diseases and Internal Medicine at Tufts New England Medical Center. Dr. Simmons received his B.S. in 1951 from the University of Pittsburgh, where he received his M.D. in 1957. In 1964 he received his M.P.H. from Harvard University.

Commission Members

Morris B. Abram, J.D., is an attorney with Paul, Weiss, Rifkind, Wharton & Garrison, New York. Mr. Abram has received Presidential appointments to advisory positions under Presidents Reagan, Carter, Johnson, and Kennedy, including Chairman of the President's Commission for the Study of Ethical Problems in Medicine and Biomedical and Behavioral Studies. He is the author of numerous articles including "Public Involvement in Medical Ethics—Model for Government Action." Mr. Abram frequently lectures before professional organizations throughout the U.S. and abroad on the subjects of Biomedical Ethics and Civil Rights. Mr. Abram received his B.A. in 1938 from the University of Georgia and in 1940 he received his J.D. degree from the University of Chicago. As a Rhodes Scholar at Oxford University, he received his B.A. in 1948, and his M.A. in 1953.

Stuart H. Altman, Ph.D., is Dean of the Florence Heller Graduate School for Social Policy and Sol C. Chaiken Professor of National Health Policy at Brandeis University. Dr. Altman also serves as Chairman of the congressionally-mandated Prospective Payment Assessment Commission, to which he was appointed in 1984 and reappointed in 1987. From

1971 to 1976, he was Deputy Assistant Secretary for Planning and Evaluation of the Department of Health, Education and Welfare (HEW). In 1973-74 he was Deputy Director for Health of the President's Cost-of-Living Council, where he was responsible for developing the Council's program on health care cost containment. He has served on the Board of the Robert Wood Johnson Clinical Scholars Program and on the Governing Council of the Institute of Medicine. He has taught at Brandeis and Brown Universities and the Graduate School of Public Policy at the University of California at Berkeley. Dr. Altman received his B.A. in Economics from City College of New York in 1959 and his M.A. in 1961 and Ph.D. in 1964, both in Economics, from the University of California at Los Angeles.

William F. Buehler is Group Vice President—Human Resources, AT&T, New Jersey. Mr. Buehler has been with AT&T since 1964. In December 1982, Mr. Buehler was named Vice President—General Business Systems. Mr. Buehler is active in many organizations, including the Alliance for Employee Growth and Development, Inc. Board of Trustees; New Jersey Executive Council; College and University Relations Executive Policy Board; and the Association for International Practical Training Board of Directors. Mr. Buehler received his B.S. degree in Industrial Engineering from Lafayette College in 1961, and attended the Wharton Advanced Marketing Program in 1976, and the Aspen Institute for Humanistic Studies in 1980.

Walton E. Burdick is Vice President—Personnel, IBM. Mr. Burdick has been with IBM since 1955. Mr. Burdick was appointed by President Reagan as a commissioner on the National Commission for Employment Policy and has served as the Chairman of the Business Roundtable's Employee Relations Committee. Mr. Burdick is a member of the National Board of Junior Achievement and the Board of Directors of the National Alliance of Business. Mr. Burdick serves as a member of the Cornell University Council where he received a B.S. degree in industrial and labor relations.

Robert Neil Butler, M.D., is the Brookdale Professor and Chairman of the Gerald and May Ellen Ritter Department of Geriatrics and Adult Development at the Mount Sinai Medical Center. Prior to 1982, Dr. Butler was Director of the National Institute on Aging with the National Institute of Health. Dr. Butler is a member of the Health Advisory Committee, Public Affairs Committee, The International Institute on Aging, and the National Edith K. Ehrman East Harlem Health Education Advisory Committee. Dr. Butler is the Co-Creator of *Lifetime Magazine* on Public Television and Editor of *Long Life Series* published by Ballantine Books.

Dr. Butler also serves as President of the Regional Committee for North America of the Sandoz Foundation for Gerontology Research. Dr. Butler received a B.A. from Columbia University in 1949 and an M.D. in 1953.

Theodore Cooper, M.D., Ph.D., is Chairman and Chief Executive Officer, The Upjohn Company. Prior to joining the Upjohn Company, Dr. Cooper was Dean of Cornell University Medical College and Provost for Medical Affairs. Dr. Cooper has served as Director of the National Heart & Lung Institute of the National Institutes of Health as well as Assistant Secretary for Health, in the Department of Health, Education and Welfare. Dr. Cooper has also served on the boards of the Metropolitan Life Insurance Company; Borden, Inc.; Harris Bankcorp, Inc., Harris Trust and Savings Bank; and Bronson Healthcare Group, Inc. Dr. Cooper earned a B.S. in 1949 from Georgetown University, an M.D. in 1954 from St. Louis University School of Medicine, and a Ph.D. in Philosophy in 1956 from St. Louis University Graduate School.

Merlin K. DuVal, M.D., is Senior Vice President, Samaritan Health Services. Dr. DuVal has served as Assistant Secretary of Health, Department of Health, Education and Welfare, and has served as chief in both the delegation to the World Health Organization, Geneva, Switzerland, and U.S. Delegation to the Western Hemisphere Ministers of Health, Santiago, Chile. Dr. DuVal is a member of the Board of Directors for Project Insure and Westberg Institute, as well as several associations, including the American Association for the Advancement of Science; American Medical Association; the Institute of Medicine (IOM), National Academy of Sciences; and the IOM Board of Health Promotion and Disease Prevention. Dr. DuVal is the author of over 100 publications, including "What's Ahead in Healthcare Legislation." Dr. DuVal earned an A.B. degree from Dartmouth, and an M.D. from Cornell University Medical College.

George C. Eads, Ph.D., is Vice President and Chief Economist of the General Motors Corporation. Prior to 1986, Dr. Eads was Dean of the School of Public Affairs at the University of Maryland, where he had been a faculty member since 1981. From 1979 to 1981, he was a member of the Council of Economic Advisors (CEA). Dr. Eads founded and directed the RAND Corporation's research program in regulatory policies and institutions. He also served as Executive Director of the National Commission on Supplies and Shortages; Assistant Director for Government Operations and Research of the Council on Wage and Price Stability; special assistant to the Assistant Attorney General of the antitrust division of the U.S. Department of Justice; and Program Manager for the National Science Foundation in Washington, D.C. He taught at the University of Maryland, Yale, Harvard, Princeton, and George Washington

Universities. Dr. Eads received his M.A. and Ph.D. in Economics from Yale University.

Charles C. Edwards, M.D., is President and Chief Executive Officer of Scripps Clinic and Research Foundation. Dr. Edwards has served as a consultant to the U.S. Public Health Service, as President of the National Health Council, and presently serves on the Board of Governors, Hospital Corporation of America; Consultant, General Accounting Office's Health Advisory Committee; and President, Board of Directors, Coordinated Healthcare System. In 1969 he was appointed by President Nixon as Commissioner of the Food and Drug Administration. Dr. Edwards earned a B.A. in 1945 and an M.D. in 1948, both from the University of Colorado.

Harry D. Garber is Vice Chairman of the Board of the Equitable Life Assurance Society of the United States. He has been with Equitable Life Assurance Society since 1950. Mr. Garber is also a Director of the Equitable Variable Life Insurance Company. He serves on the boards of Genesco, Inc., the American Women's Economic Development Corporation and is currently a member of the Board of Trustees of Howard University. Mr. Garber is actively involved in the federal legislation and tax arenas. In 1950, Mr. Garber received a B.A. from Yale University.

Robert H. Gaynor is Group Vice President–Planning, AT&T Communications (retired). Prior to 1986, Mr. Gaynor was Vice President–Personnel, AT&T Communications. Mr. Gaynor served on the Board of Directors of AT&T Communications and American Transtech. Mr. Gaynor was Vice Chairman of the Chamber of Commerce of Greater Kansas City and served as a trustee of the University of Missouri, where he is presently Chairman of the Board of Visitors and Special Consultant to the Chancellor. He serves as Vice Chairman of Inroads, Inc. (assisting minority people through college and into leadership positions) and on the National Executive Board of the Boy Scouts of America. While serving in the military Mr. Gaynor received a B.S. degree from the University of Michigan in 1946. He has attended the University of Pennsylvania's Institute of Humanistic Studies and studied advanced communications at Dartmouth College.

J. Peter Grace is Chairman, President and Chief Executive Officer of W.R. Grace & Company. Mr. Grace has been with W.R. Grace & Company since 1936. He has served as an adviser to three Presidents: Eisenhower, Kennedy, and most recently was appointed by President Reagan in 1982 as Chairman of the President's Private Sector Survey on Cost Control in Federal Government. Mr. Grace is the author of a book entitled *Burning Money: The Waste of Your Tax Dollar*. Mr. Grace is a member of the Council on Foreign Relations; founding member of the Emergency Committee for American Trade; and a member of the Development Committee of the National Bureau of Economic Research, Inc. He has received several honorary degrees and received the Jefferson Award for the Greater Public Service by a private citizen from the American Institute for Public Service. Mr. Grace is a 1936 Yale graduate.

Sister Mary Corita Heid, R.S.M., is President of the Sisters of Mercy Health Corporation. Sister Heid is presently a member of the Mercy Systems Board of Directors, Mercy Services for the Aging Board of Directors, and the Mercy Health Services Board of Directors. She is also a member of the Board of Trustees, Sister of Mercy Health Corporation. Sister Heid has received the Outstanding Woman in Business Award, as well as the YMCA Achievement Award for Professions. Sister Mary Corita Heid entered the Novitiate of the Sisters of Mercy in 1957. She received a B.S. in nursing in 1963 from Mercy College and an M.A. in Hospital and Health Administration in 1970 from the University of Iowa.

J. Bruce Johnston, J.D., is Executive Vice President–Employee Relations, USX Corporation. Mr. Johnston is a member of USX's Policy Committee. He has served as chief labor negotiator for the steel, coal, cement, maritime and construction industries. Mr. Johnston is a director of Equibank Corporation, a director of the National Association of Manufacturers, a member of the Business Roundtable, and chairs the International Iron and Steel Institute's Industrial Relations Committee. Mr. Johnston also serves as trustee with United States Steel & Carnegie Pension Fund, Robert Morris College, Children's Hospital of Pittsburgh, and WQED Public Television. Mr. Johnston graduated from the University of Pittsburgh with a B.A. and J.D.

Reverend Paul F. McCleary is Executive Director of the Christian Children's Fund. Prior to his appointment as Executive Director, Rev. McCleary served as Executive Vice President and Acting President of Save the Children. Rev. McCleary has also served as Associate General Secretary for research of the General Council on Ministries of the United Methodist Church, and for nine years as the Executive Director of Church World Service and Associate Secretary for the Division on Overseas Ministries of the National Council of Churches of Christ. Rev. McCleary serves as a member of several committees, including the Committee on African Development Strategies of the Overseas Development Council and the Council on Foreign Relations; and the World Future Society. During 1988, Rev. McCleary has been particularly active as Co-Chairman of InterAction and in his effort to reforge the International Save the Children Alliance. Rev. McCleary received a B.A in 1952 from Olivet Nazarene College, an M.Div. from Garrett Theological Seminary in 1956, and an M.A. in 1972 from Northwestern University.

John Alexander McMahon, J.D., is Chairman, Department of Health Administration, at Duke University. Prior to joining Duke University, Mr. McMahon served as President of the American Hospital Association. In 1968, Mr. McMahon became the first President of Blue Cross and Blue Shield of North Carolina. Mr. McMahon is Chairman-Emeritus of the Board of Duke University. He is a member of the Institute of Medicine of the National Academy of Sciences and of the North Carolina Institute of Medicine. In 1942, Mr. McMahon earned an A.B. from Duke University. Mr. McMahon attended Harvard Business School from 1942 through 1943 and in 1948 received a J.D. from Harvard Law School.

Richard J. Merrill, LL.B., is a professor and formerly the Dean of the University of Virginia Law School. Mr. Merrill has served as Chief Counsel to the U.S. Food and Drug Administration. Mr. Merrill has been a member of the Council of the Institute of Medicine, National Academy of Sciences (NAS) since 1977. He is also a member of the Environmental Protection Agency's (EPA) Biotechnology Science Advisory Committee. Mr. Merrill has served as a member of EPA Administrator's Advisory Committee, NAS Committee on Institutional Means for Risk Assessment, and as a consultant to the Office of Technology Assessment of the U.S. Congress and to the Office of Science and Technology Policy of the Executive Office of the President. Mr. Merrill is the author of several books and articles, including *Food and Drug Law: Case and Materials,* and *Risk Quantitation and Regulatory Policy: Banbury Report 19.* In 1959, Mr. Merrill received an A.B. from Columbia College. As a Rhodes Scholar, Mr. Merrill received a B.A. and an M.A. from Oxford University in 1961 and went on to receive an LL.B. from Columbia University School of Law, where he was Editor-in-Chief of the *Columbia Law Review.*

Edmund D. Pellegrino, M.D., is Director of the Kennedy Institute of Ethics at Georgetown University and a John Carroll Professor of Medicine and Medical Humanities at Georgetown University Medical Center. Prior to his appointment at Georgetown University, Dr. Pellegrino was President of The Catholic University of America, and earlier the President and Chairman of the Board of Directors of Yale–New Haven Medical Center, Inc., as well as a Professor of Medicine at Yale University School of Medicine. Dr. Pellegrino is currently a member of over thirty committees and boards including Board of Directors of the International Hospice Institute, a member of the National Advisory Council on Health Care Technology Assessment, and a Member of the American College of Physicians Ethics Committee. He has served as President of the Society for Health and Human Values, and as Chairman of the Medical Advisory Committee, The Network for Continuing Medical Education. Dr. Pellegrino is the author of articles on medicine, medical education and philosophy, scientific articles, books, abstracts and book reviews totaling over 400. Dr. Pellegrino received a B.S. from St. John's University in 1941 and an M.D. from New York University College of Medicine.

Douglas S. Peters is Senior Vice President of Representation and Public Affairs for Blue Cross and Blue Shield Association. Prior to joining Blue Cross and Blue Shield, Mr. Peters was President and Chief Executive Officer of the Henry Ford Hospital and Executive Vice President of the Henry Ford Health Care Corporation. Mr. Peters has served on the board of the Michigan Hospital Association and on several committees of the American Hospital Association. He is a fellow in the American College of Healthcare Executives. Mr. Peters served as the Director of the University of Nebraska Hospital and Clinics, and as an associate director of the University of Michigan Hospitals. Mr. Peters received a B.S. degree from Ohio State University in 1965 and an M.A. degree in Hospital Administration at the University of Michigan in 1967.

Jane C. Pfeiffer is a management consultant in the areas of management organization, communications and government relations. Mrs. Pfeiffer has served as Chairman of the Board of the National Broadcasting Company. Prior to joining NBC, Mrs. Pfeiffer had a twenty-year career with IBM, leaving as Vice President of Communications and Government Relations. Mrs. Pfeiffer serves as director of Ashland Oil, Inc., International Paper Company, and J.C. Penney Company. She is a trustee of the University of Notre Dame and the Overseas Development Council and is a member of the Council on Foreign Relations and the Economic Club. Mrs. Pfeiffer has been a member of several government commissions, including the President's Commission on White House Fellows, the General Advisory Committee on Arms Control and Disarmament, and the President's Commission on Military Compensation.

Uwe E. Reinhardt, Ph.D., is James Madison Professor of Political Economy at Princeton University's Woodrow Wilson School of Public and International Affairs, where he has taught since 1968. Dr. Reinhardt currently serves on the Committee on the Implications of For-Profit Medicine at the Institute of Medicine, National Academy of Sciences, and on the Physician Payment Review Commission (PPRC). From 1979 to 1981, he served on the Department of Health, Education and Welfare's National Health Care Technology Council, and in 1981 he became a member of the Department of Health and Human Services' Private Sector Task Force on Health Policy. Dr. Reinhardt also served on the Veterans Administration's Special Medical Advisory Group and the Editorial Boards of *Health and Society, Health Affairs, Patient Care, Health Policy and Education,* and *The Journal of Health Economics.* In 1964, Dr. Reinhardt received a Bachelors of Commerce with honors in Economics from the University of Saskatchewan. Dr. Reinhardt received his M.A. and Ph.D. in Economics from Yale University.

Alice M. Rivlin, Ph.D., is a senior fellow and former Director of the Economic Studies Program of The Brookings Institution. Dr. Rivlin was the first Director of the Congressional Budget Office. She has also served as Assistant Secretary for Planning and Evaluation in the U.S. Department of Health, Education and Welfare. In 1988, she was a visiting Professor at the Kennedy School of Government at Harvard University. Dr. Rivlin is the author of numerous books and articles on the U.S. economy, the budget, and public decisionmaking, including *Caring for the Disabled Elderly, Systematic Thinking for Social Action,* and editor of *Economic Choices 1984.* She is the recipient of the MacArthur Foundation Fellowship and was Harvard's Godkin Lecturer in 1984. Dr. Rivlin was the President of the American Economic Association in 1986 and is currently a Director of the Unisys Corporation and the Union Carbide Corporation. Dr. Rivlin graduated from Bryn Mawr College in 1952 and received a Ph.D. in Economics from Radcliffe in 1958.

Charles S. Robb, J.D., Senator from Virginia, was an attorney with Hunton & Williams. Mr. Robb served as Governor of the State of Virginia from 1982 to 1986. During his term as Governor, Mr. Robb served on numerous committees, including Chairman of the Southern Governor's Association, Chairman of the Democratic Governor's Association, Chairman of the Education Commission of the States, and President of the Council of State Governments. Mr. Robb served on several boards, including Crestar Financial Corporation, The Carnegie Foundation for the Advancement of Teaching, the Enterprise Foundation, The Coalition for Democratic Majority, and the National Commission on the Public Service. Mr. Robb received his B.A. from the University of Wisconsin in 1961 and in 1973 he received his law degree from the University of Virginia.

C. B. Rogers, Jr., is President and COO, Equifax, Inc. Prior to joining Equifax Mr. Rogers was Senior Vice President of Corporate Services Staffs for International Business Machines Corporation where he served as a member of IBM's Corporate Management Board and the Management Committee. Mr. Rogers serves on many boards, including Sears Roebuck and Company, IBM World Trade Asia/Pacific Group, MCI and Equifax, Inc. In addition, he is a member of the Board of Visitors at Duke University School of Business and a trustee of Greenwich Academy. Mr. Rogers is a graduate of Gettysburg College. He received his M.B.A. degree from George Washington University.

David E. Rogers, M.D., is the Walsh McDermott University Professor of Medicine at Cornell University Medical College. For the 15 years prior to this appointment, Dr. Rogers was the President of the Robert Wood Johnson Foundation. Dr. Rogers has served as Dean of Medicine and Vice President for Medical Affairs at Johns Hopkins University and Medical Director of The Johns Hopkins Hospital. He is a member of numerous medical societies and organizations, including the Scientific Advisory Board of Scripps Clinic and Research Foundation; Institute of Medicine, National Academy of Sciences; and has served as Chairman of the Council on Foundations and as President of the Association of American Physicians. Dr. Rogers is the author of over 200 scientific publications and has been the editor of *The Year Book of Medicine* since 1966. Dr. Rogers attended Ohio State University from 1942 to 1944 and Miami University of Ohio in 1944. He received his M.D. from Cornell University Medical College in 1948.

James B. Rogers, Jr., is Chairman of Rogers Holdings and a Professor, Columbia University Graduate School of Business. From 1973 through 1980, Mr. Rogers was Executive Vice President of Soros Fund Management. Mr. Rogers was an Investment Analyst for both Arnold and S. Bleichroader, Inc., and Bache and Company. Mr. Rogers was Assistant Chairman of the Board, Neuberger and Berman, Inc. In 1964 Mr. Rogers received a B.A. in History from Yale University and in 1966, a B.A. and M.A. from Balliol College at Oxford University.

Jill S. Ruckelshaus serves on the Board of Directors for the Women's Campaign Fund. Prior to 1983, Mrs. Ruckelshaus was Commissioner of the U.S. Commission on Civil Rights. She has served as Vice President of the National Center for Voluntary Action and as a delegate to the United Nations Conference on Women in Mexico City. Mrs. Ruckelshaus has served as Assistant to the President for Women's Affairs. Currently, Mrs. Ruckelshaus is Chairman of the Washington World Affairs Fellows while serving as a trustee for the Lakeside School, the University of Puget Sound, and the Institute for Resource Management. She also serves on the Board of Directors for Sea-First Bank, Lincoln National Corporation, Washington Women's Education Foundation, Peabody Award Advisory Board, and Northwest Education Foundation. She is a member of the Commission for African Development and the Hitachi Foundation Advisory Board.

James H. Sammons, M.D., is Executive Vice President of the American Medical Association (AMA). Prior to becoming chief executive officer of the AMA in 1974, Dr. Sammons conducted an active private family practice in Baytown, Texas, and was clinical assistant professor at Baylor University College of Medicine. Dr. Sammons is a member of numerous commissions and boards, including The Institute of Medicine, General Motors Medical Committee for Automotive Safety, the Department of

Health and Human Services Private/Public Sector Advisory Committee on Catastrophic Illness, the Dunlop Group of Six, and the Board of Directors of Friends of the National Library of Medicine. Dr. Sammons served for 11 years on the Texas Medical Association (TMA) Board of Councilors, and was its chairman for 3 years. He was also a member of the TMA Judicial Council, TMA Executive Board and was TMA President. Dr. Sammons completed his premedical studies at Washington and Lee University, and received his M.D. degree from St. Louis University School of Medicine in 1951.

David Satcher, M.D., Ph.D., is President of Meharry Medical College. Prior to joining Meharry in 1982, Dr. Satcher was professor and chairman of the Department of Community Medicine of the School of Medicine at Morehouse College. Dr. Satcher serves on the Board of Directors of Friends of the National Library of Medicine and the Robert Wood Johnson Clinical Scholars Programs. Recently, Dr. Satcher was appointed Vice-Chairman of the Council on Graduate Medical Education. He serves as a Diplomate of the American Board of Family Practice and a Fellow of the American Academy of Family Physicians. Dr. Satcher received his undergraduate degree from Morehouse College and went on to receive his M.D. and Ph.D. from Case Western Reserve University.

John J. Sweeney is President of the Service Employees International Union, AFL-CIO, CLC. Mr. Sweeney was first elected in 1980 and was recently elected to a third four-year term as president. Prior to 1980, Mr. Sweeney had been secretary-treasurer of the union. He has also served as vice president of the New York City Central Labor Council. Sweeney is a board member of the American Arbitration Association, the American Red Cross, the Catholic Youth Organization, and the Citizen-Labor Energy Coalition. He is on the labor advisory board of American Income Life Insurance Company Program for Affordable Health Care. In 1987 he co-edited the UNA-USA Economic Policy Council's *Family and Work: Bridging the Gap*. Mr. Sweeney received a degree in economics from Iona College.

Samuel O. Thier, M.D., is the President of the Institute of Medicine, National Academy of Sciences. Prior to his appointment, Dr. Thier was Sterling Professor and Chairman of the Department of Internal Medicine at Yale University School of Medicine. He has served as president of the American Federation of Clinical Research, Mexican College of Physicians, and Chairman, American Board of Internal Medicine. From 1980 to 1984, Dr. Thier served on the Director's Advisory Committee with the National Institutes of Health. Dr. Thier is the author of numerous articles on renal physiology and has co-authored with his colleague Lloyd H. Smith, Jr., M.D., *Pathophysiology, The Biological Principles of Disease*. Dr.

Thier received his undergraduate degree from Cornell University in 1956 and his M.D. from State University of New York at Syracuse in 1960.

COMMISSION ADVISERS

David Banta, M.D., is in the Department of Health Economics, Faculty of Medicine, State University of Limburg, The Netherlands. He is the former Director of the Health Section for the Office of Technology Assessment of the U.S. Congress.

Steven C. Beering, M.D., is President of Purdue University. Prior to his appointment at Purdue, Dr. Beering was Dean of the University of Indiana School of Medicine.

Charles R. Buck, Jr., Sc.D., is the Staff Executive of the Health Care Programs for General Electric Company. Prior to joining General Electric Company, Mr. Buck was the Executive Director of the University of Pennsylvania Hospital.

Roger Bulger, M.D., is the President of the Association of Academic Health Centers. Dr. Bulger was President of the University of Texas Health Science Center before he joined the AAHC.

Guido Calabresi, LL.B., is the Dean of Yale University Law School. Prior to joining Yale Law School he was the Dean of Columbia Law School.

Thomas Chalmers, M.D., is Distinguished Physician at the Boston Veterans Administration Medical Center. Mr. Chalmers has served as the President and Dean of the Mount Sinai Medical Center in New York.

The Honorable Clark Clifford, J.D., an attorney with Clifford & Warnke, is a long-time presidential adviser.

William Foege, M.D., is the Executive Director of the Task Force of Child Survival at the Carter Center, Emory University. Formerly, Dr. Foege served as the Director for the Centers for Disease Control.

Rev. Theodore M. Hesburgh, C.S.C., is President Emeritus of the University of Notre Dame. Reverend Hesburgh was awarded the Cardinal Gibbons Medal from Catholic University. He serves as a trustee to the Committee on Foreign Relations.

The Honorable Carla Hills, LL.B., is the United States Trade Representative. She was Co-managing Partner of Weil, Gotshal & Manges. Ms. Hill is a former Secretary of the Department of Housing and Urban Development under President Ford.

John Hogness, M.D., has served as the President of the Association of Academic Health Centers and as the President of the University of Washington.

The Honorable Barbara Jordan, J.D., is a Professor at the L.B.J. School of Public Affairs, University of Texas. Ms. Jordan is also a former congresswoman from Texas, serving in the 93rd through 95th Congresses.

Michael Maccoby, Ph.D., is the Director of the Program on Technology, Public Policy & Human Development of the John F. Kennedy School of Government at Harvard University. Dr. Maccoby is a consultant to business, government, and unions, as well as an author of numerous publications including *The Leader*.

Catherine E. McDermott is the President of Grant Makers in Health. Ms. McDermott has also worked for the Robert Wood Johnson Foundation.

Dennis O'Leary, M.D., is the President of the Joint Commission on Accreditation of Healthcare Organizations.

Paul H. O'Neill is the Chairman and Chief Executive Officer of the Aluminum Company of America. Mr. O'Neill has served as President of International Paper Company and as Deputy Director of the Office of Management and Budget for the White House.

Robert G. Petersdorf, M.D., is President of the Association of American Medical Colleges. Prior to his appointment as AAMC President, Dr. Petersdorf was Vice-Chancellor for Health Sciences and Dean at the University of California San Diego School of Medicine.

Arnold S. Relman, M.D., is the Editor-in-Chief of the *New England Journal of Medicine*.

The Honorable Elliot Richardson, LL.B., is an attorney with Milbank, Tweed, Hadley & McCloy. Mr. Richardson is a former secretary of the Department of Health, Education and Welfare.

Lewis Thomas, M.D., is President Emeritus of the Memorial Sloan-Kettering Cancer Center and the well-known author of *Lives of a Cell*.

⌐⌐ ⌐⌐

Appendix B

⌐⌐ ⌐⌐

Commission Meetings and Expert Witnesses

MEETINGS OF THE FULL COMMISSION

October 3, 1986
First Commission meeting. Approval of charter, press release, and focus on the three major topics of accessibility, cost, and quality of health care.

January 12, 1987
Second Commission meeting. Discussion of the nature and magnitude of the problems in access, cost, and quality of health care. Presentation of the Canadian health care system by Canadian economist Robert Evans.

April 2, 1987
Third Commission meeting. Discussion of the style and content of a draft interim report detailing the problems in the health care system.

WORKSHOPS

July 7, 1987
"Promoting Personal Responsibility for Health"

September 29, 1987
"Improving Access to Care for the Medically Indigent: Examining Options for the Uninsured"

November 17, 1987
"How Can We Improve the Appropriateness and Effectiveness of Medical Care?"

January 14-15, 1988
"How Can We Improve Quality Management?"

February 9, 1988
"How Can We Develop an Adequate Level of Care?"

February 10, 1988   "Financing Long-Term Care for the Elderly: Public and Private Options"

March 18, 1988   "How Can We Control Costs and Optimize Efficiency?"

RETREATS

April 28-30, 1988

July 6-7, 1988

September 29-30,
1988

EXPERT WITNESSES

Meetings

October 3, 1986   Daniel Callahan, Ph.D.
                        The Hastings Center

                        Kathy Lohr, Ph.D.
                        Institute of Medicine
                        (In 1986—The RAND Corporation)

                        Gail Wilensky, Ph.D.
                        Project HOPE

January 12, 1986   Professor Robert G. Evans
                        University of British Columbia

Workshops

July 7, 1987   *Promoting Personal Responsibility for Health*

                        Walter Anderson
                        Regional Sales Director
                        Johnson & Johnson Health Management

                        Gordon H. DeFriese, Ph.D.
                        Director, Health Services Research Center
                        University of North Carolina

                        Dorothea Johnson, M.D.
                        Corporate Vice-President for Health Affairs
                        AT&T

Marshall Kreuter, Ph.D.
Director, Division of Health Education
Centers for Disease Control

Robert S. Lawrence, M.D.
Director, Department of Medicine
Cambridge Hospital

J. Michael McGinnis
Deputy Assistant Secretary for Health, HHS

June Osborn, M.D.
Dean, University of Michigan School of Public
  Health

Marian Osterweis, Ph.D.
Institute of Medicine

Louise Russell, Ph.D.
Rutgers University
(in 1987—The Brookings Institution)

Robert M. Veatch, Ph.D.
Kennedy Institute of Ethics, Georgetown
  University

September 29, 1987   *Improving Access to Care for the Medically Indigent:*
                      Examining Options for the Uninsured

Randall Bovbjerg
The Urban Institute

Deborah J. Chollet, Ph.D.
Employee Benefit Research Institute

Robert Crittenden, M.D.
School of Public Health, University of
  Washington

Richard E. Curtis
National Governors' Association

Karen Ignagni
AFL/CIO

Debra J. Lipson
Intergovernmental Health Policy Project
George Washington University

David Nexon
U.S. Senate Committee on Labor and Human
    Resources

Frank S. Swain
U.S. Small Business Administration

November 17, 1987   *How Can We Improve the Appropriateness and Effec-
                        tiveness of Medical Care?*

Robert H. Brook, M.D.
The RAND Corporation

David Eddy, M.D.
Director, Center for Health Policy Research and
    Education, Duke University

George D. Lundberg, M.D.
Editor, *Journal of the American Medical Association*

Arnold S. Relman, M.D.
Editor-in-Chief, *New England Journal of Medicine*

January 14-15, 1988   *How Can We Improve Quality Management?*

Donald M. Berwick, M.D.
Harvard Community Health Plan

Otis Bowen, M.D.
Secretary, Department of Health and Human
    Services

Kathryn Boyer, C.N.M.
Former President, American College of
    Nurse-Midwives Foundation

Leo P. Brideau
Strong Memorial Hospital

Robert H. Brook, M.D.
The RAND Corporation

John M. Eisenberg, M.D.
Hospital of the University of Pennsylvania

Harvey V. Fineberg, M.D.
Dean, Harvard School of Public Health

Palma E. Formica, M.D.
President, New Jersey Medical Society

Harry S. Jonas, M.D.
Director, Division of Undergraduate Medical
Education, American Medical Association

Dennis O'Leary, M.D.
President, Joint Commission on Accreditation
of Healthcare Organizations

Jack W. Owen
Executive Vice President
American Hospital Association

David N. Sundwall, M.D.
Administrator
Health Resources and Services Administration

Walter J. Wadlington, J.D.
University of Virginia Law School

Douglas P. Wagner, Ph.D.
George Washington University Medical Center

Andrew H. Webber
Executive Vice President
American Medical Peer Review Association

Sidney M. Wolfe, M.D.
Director, Public Citizen Health Research Group

February 9, 1988   *How Can We Develop an Adequate Level of Care?*

Diane B. McCarthy
Health Policy Agenda

Governor Scott M. Matheson
Health Policy Agenda

February 10, 1988   *Financing Long-Term Care for the Elderly: Public and
                          Private Options*

Daniel P. Bourque
Corporate Senior Vice President
Voluntary Hospitals of America

Bruce L. Boyd
Chairman, HIAA Long-Term Care Task Force

Stephen R. McConnell, Ph.D.
Coordinator, Long-Term Care '88

John C. Rother, J.D.
American Association of Retired Persons

Anne R. Somers
Robert Wood Johnson Medical School

Joshua M. Wiener, Ph.D.
The Brookings Institution

March 18, 1988   *How Can We Control Costs and Optimize Efficiency?*

Beach B. Hall
General Motors Corporation

Lawrence S. Lewin
President, Lewin/ICF, Incorporated

Retreat

April 28-30, 1988   Donald M. Berwick, M.D.
Harvard Community Health Plan

Robert H. Brook, M.D.
The RAND Corporation

⌐ ⌐
Appendix C
⌐ ⌐

Examples of Current Quality Improvement Activities

A National Quality Improvement Initiative would provide a broad vision coordinating and expanding important ongoing activities including, but certainly not limited to: the Effectiveness Initiative of The Department of Health and Human Services (HHS), the Patient Outcomes Assessment Research Program of the National Center for Health Services Research and Health Care Technology Assessment (NCHSR), the American Medical Association's (AMA) quality agenda, Institute of Medicine's (IOM) national technology assessment program of the Council on Health Care Technology, the Agenda for Change of the Joint Commission on Accreditation of Healthcare Organizations (JCAHO), and the many academic centers already under contract with these and other programs.

The Commission heard from experts involved in these and many other efforts. The examples provided in this appendix represent only a small sampling of those currently in existence.

TECHNOLOGY ASSESSMENT AND APPROPRIATENESS RESEARCH

How much do we know about our technology? Technology is used here to mean all the medical and surgical procedures, drugs, tools, and instruments doctors use to prevent, diagnose, and treat disease. Appropriate health care is that which is deemed effective for the condition for which it is provided, as measured by solid technology assessment, of whether it is appropriate both in general and in actual situations. Predetermined criteria for specific appropriateness may include such factors as impact on functional well-being, degree of efficiency, or conformance to a societal goal such as equity of access to a particular technology.

While a good deal of research is conducted on various medical technologies, not enough has been done on their effectiveness in common settings or in very specific circumstances. In other words, whether a technology works does not necessarily answer the question whether it makes a difference in the end result.

Dr. Robert H. Brook, a pioneering researcher in the quality of health care, described a system he envisions for linking the field of quality with that of technology assessment:

> The final system might operate in the following way: A technology assessment is performed. Its conclusions are then integrated into data banks containing information from previous technology assessments. This step most likely requires additional quantitative analyses. Once these are completed, the new, augmented information replaces the old in models that are used to generate quality-of-care criteria or standards. The results of this effort are presented to a series of experts for their review, revision, and approval. Finally, the ensuing quality-of-care standards and criteria, along with the analysis supporting their use, are made available to organizations or agencies charged with the business of quality assessment. (1)

Activities are underway that address pieces of Dr. Brook's vision. As a starting point, in late October 1988, at the request of the Health Care Financing Administration, the Institute of Medicine convened a panel of thirteen leading physicians to select conditions in need of more rigorous assessment. The panel members selected treatment of angina pectoris (chest pain), heart attacks, strokes, breast cancer, prostate problems, and hip fractures. A number of considerations can affect priority selections, including: the amount of dollars they cost the government (and the taxpayers) every year, how often the procedure is done, the number of people potentially affected by the technology, and the technology's stage of development at the time of the assessment.

The RAND Corporation has spent the last several years measuring the appropriateness of a number of specific medical and surgical procedures. They have applied this process and, in a 1986 study on the "Variations in the Use of Medical and Surgical Services by the Medicare Population," found that "of the 123 procedures studied, 67 showed at least threefold differences between sites with the highest and lowest rates of use." (2) In 1987 the RAND researchers published the results of another study in which they examined the appropriateness of use of three procedures—coronary angiography, carotid endarterectomy, and upper gastrointestinal tract endoscopy. The researchers concluded that "differences in appropriateness cannot explain geographic variations in the use of the procedures." (3) This kind of work looks promising, and the Commission recommends that it be continued and expanded to include additional tests and procedures.

CLINICAL TRIALS

While there have been some excellent recent trials on treatments such as coronary artery bypass surgery or on alternative breast cancer treatments, the Commission recommends encouraging more clinical trials as new technologies, especially procedures, are developed. Making the best decisions requires having the best evidence available, and we simply do not do enough trials as new technologies are developed. We need to orient more trials toward long-term outcomes. Trials should include the collection of cost information, so that appropriate payment related to the resource costs of the technology can be established as soon as a new technology enters the system, with an explicit understanding that the resource costs are likely to change as the technology's use becomes more widespread.

RESEARCH ON METHODS

Several of the methodologies used in research on quality and appropriateness need refinement. Although a number of efforts are currently in progress, they are not enough. The Commission endorses much of the work already underway in this area; it considers the following research[1] critical and urges that it be continued:

- Dr. David Eddy analyzes the quality of medical evidence and its use in medical practice. He examines practices that are generally regarded as worthwhile and asks: What do we actually know about their effects? He presents evidence that for at least some medical practices (e.g., the treatment of glaucoma), available evidence about their effectiveness, risks, and costs is incomplete. Further, he finds for some practices, the effects are either not known or are known to be negative. (4)
- The RAND Corporation has developed a method that draws on available evidence to measure appropriateness. This method is based on consensus panels; it has been subjected to some rigorous evaluation, but it needs to be refined further. (5)(6)
- The Health Care Financing Administration is currently involved in several important areas. Some of HCFA's work includes analyses of the best use of hospital morbidity/mortality data as it re-

---

[1]Again, this does not represent a complete listing on all the research currently underway. It is meant to highlight a few examples.

lates to quality measurement, as well as analyses of different measures of severity of illness. There has been a great deal of controversy over the recently released HCFA hospital mortality data, particularly concerning their use as a method to identify poor quality care. For example, recent research indicates that, "inpatient death rates depend on length-of-stay patterns and give a biased picture of mortality." (7) Other researchers have concluded that "comorbidity must be taken into account in any prediction of hospital mortality rates to avoid misleading statements about the quality of care." (8)

- The National Center for Health Services Research, under its Patient Outcomes Assessment Research Program, is supporting the study of the usefulness of insurance claims data for evaluating outcomes, the usefulness of Connecticut's statewide data system for identifying and analyzing reasons for variations in hospital use, and the development of better techniques for analyzing and synthesizing medical literature on alternative treatment methods. (9)

- The JCAHO, a voluntary organization that accredits most of the hospitals as well as other health care organizations in the country, is developing a system to evaluate the outcomes of an organization's clinical performance through the use of clinical indicators. Examples of these outcome indicators under study include death, hospital-acquired infection, and adverse drug reactions. This groundbreaking work is attempting to establish a relationship between how we provide care and what happens as a result. The National Leadership Commission supports this and other endeavors relating quality standards to outcomes.

- In addition to these and many other efforts, the Commission urges new efforts to find ways to measure the quality of care provided outside the hospital. With today's financial incentives shifting more and more health care to outpatient settings, the need for quality assurance is obvious. The Commission is encouraged by the active involvement of the JCAHO in this area and sees a potential role for both JCAHO and Medicare's Peer Review Organizations.

OUTCOMES ASSESSMENT AND PRACTICE PATTERN MONITORING

Gaps in our knowledge add to uncertainty, and too much uncertainty leads to major variation in clinical practice. Because of these basic system flaws, many current practice standards are unsupported by adequate scientific evidence.

Fortunately, Dr. John Wennberg at the Dartmouth Medical School and his colleagues have developed a method—referred to as outcomes research—to assess the long-term outcomes of various treatments. (10) The method begins with statistical analyses of claims data bases to identify problems for further survey and analysis. For outcomes research—used here to mean the comparison of competing treatments based on a long-term evaluation of functional well-being—the Commission supports the full funding of NCHSR's Patient Outcome Assessment Research Program, authorized $20 million in FY 90 and $30 million in FY 91; it also supports NCHSR's more general proposed program, the National Program for the Assessment of Patient Outcomes.

One of the key elements of assessing outcomes is continual monitoring of medical practices. While many insurers and researchers have been conducting some analyses, the Commission recommends an increase in monitoring activities. One good example of this type of activity is the HCFA-funded research project being conducted by the Maine Medical Assessment Project and the American Medical Review Research Center (AMRRC).[2] This project applies small area analysis techniques to Medicare data and uses selected Peer Review Organizations for the dissemination of the findings. These results will be reported to physicians through educational programs. (11)

DEVELOPING NATIONAL PRACTICE GUIDELINES

Clearly practice guidelines currently exist in our medical care system. Organizations that have taken the lead in developing guidelines (though they may not call them guidelines) include many medical specialty societies, the Blue Cross and Blue Shield Association, the American Medical Association, the American College of Physicians, the Council of Medical Specialty Societies, the Joint Commission on Accreditation of Healthcare Organizations, and the National Institutes of Health. Many of these groups and others also sponsor clinical guideline-setting programs.

What are these guidelines that have been the focus of so much recent discussion?[3] Very generally, they are statements describing spe-

---

[2]AMRRC is the research affiliate of the American Medical Peer Review Association (AMPRA). AMPRA is the national association on physician-directed medical review organizations, including the federally designated Peer Review Organizations.

[3]Many of the ideas the Commission has discussed on this subject are synthesized in a recent essay by Dr. Mark Chassin. (12) The Commission has borrowed from his essay here.

cific diagnostic or therapeutic procedures that should or should not be performed in specific clinical circumstances. Guidelines can also define several levels of quality of care, from the best attainable to a minimum below which care is unacceptably poor. They can be applied to groups of patients as well as to individuals.

Guidelines can address all the general problems in quality of care, which fall into three categories: problems caused by overuse, underuse, and improper use of health care services. Traditionally, guidelines and standards have focused on the second and third categories.

What characteristics will assure that guidelines will achieve their goal of improving the practice of medicine and the health of people? They must be well constructed, reflect a consensus on clinical content, possess scientific or professional credibility, and be written in clear and unambiguous language.

Guidelines have been most effectively used when they are based on data on physician performance used in conjunction with clinical information underlying the guideline. The intervention that conveys all of this information should be focused on a narrow topic, conducted face-to-face, and delivered by a respected physician or other appropriate health care professional. The most effective interventions are followed by reinforcement, feedback, and additional data on performance.

Today too many guidelines fail to meet these characteristics. In too many cases—although there are some notable exceptions—the process by which guidelines are established has been haphazard and the evidence supporting them weak. The purpose of the National Quality Improvement Initiative is to encourage the profession to introduce some rationality into the current process, improve the validity of guidelines, improve dissemination and education, and thereby encourage the development of more effective quality assurance mechanisms.

REFERENCES

1. Brook, R., "Quality Assessment and Technology Assessment: Critical Linkages," *Quality of Care and Technology Assessment: Report of a Forum of the Council on Health Care Technology*, Institute of Medicine, National Academy Press, Washington, DC, 1988, p. 27.
2. Chassin, M., Brook, R., et al., "Variations in the Use of Medical and Surgical Services by the Medicare Population," *NEJM* 314(5):285–290, January 30, 1986.
3. Chassin, M., Kosecoff, J., et al., "Does Inappropriate Use Explain Geographic Variations in the Use of Health Care Services?" *JAMA* 258(18):2533–2537, November 13, 1987.
4. Eddy, D., and Billings, J., "The Quality of Medical Evidence and Practice," a paper produced for the National Leadership Commission on Health Care, May 1987.

5. Kosecoff, J., et al., "Obtaining Clinical Data on the Appropriateness of Medical Care in Community Practice," *JAMA* 258(18):2538–2542, November 13, 1987.

6. Chassin, M., Kosecoff, J., et al., "How Coronary Angiography is Used," *JAMA* 258(18):2543–2545, November 13, 1987.

7. Jencks, S., Williams, D., and Kay, T., "Assessing Hospital-Associated Deaths from Discharge Data: The Role of Length of Stay and Comorbidities," *JAMA* 260(15):2240–2246, October 21, 1988.

8. Greenfield, S., Aronow, H., et al., "Flaws in Mortality Data: The Hazards of Ignoring Comorbid Disease," *JAMA* 260(15):2253–2255, October 21, 1988.

9. Fitzmaurice, J., Director, National Center for Health Services Research, personal communication to Dr. M. Rhoades, December 30, 1988.

10. Wennberg, J., testimony before the U.S. Senate Committee on Finance, Subcommittee on Health, July 11, 1988.

11. Webber, A., testimony before the U.S. Senate Committee on Finance, Subcommittee on Health, July 11, 1988.

12. Chassin, M., *Standards of Care in Medicine,* prepared for the Health Industry Manufacturers' Association Health Policy Seminar, Woods Hole, MA, August 1988, p. 18.

⌐⌐ ⌐⌐

Appendix D

⌐⌐ ⌐⌐

The Lewin/ICF Health Benefits Simulation Model[1]

The Health Benefits Simulation Model (HBSM) simulates the impact of changes in the eligibility, coverage, and benefits provisions of public and private health plans on households and total health benefit payments from various sources (Medicaid, employer plans, out-of-pocket, etc.). In this study, the model was used to estimate changes in household out-of-pocket health care expenditures and changes in household premium payments resulting from the illustrative plans described in Appendix E. The model was also used to estimate expenditures under the illustrative plan and fee rates required to finance the UNAC program proposed by the Commission. The model simulated the impact of these policy alternatives on selected demographic groups and the aggregate impact of the Commission's plan on total payments by public and private insurers.

A. Data Base

The HBSM is based on the 1980 National Medical Care Utilization and Expenditure Survey (NMCUES). The NMCUES provides detailed information on demographic and economic characteristics, sources of health care coverage, number and types of health care contacts during 1980, and charges by source of payment for each health care contact during that year for a sample of about 17,000 persons (6,000 households).

We adjusted these data to reflect changes in population, real incomes and other economic conditions, health care utilization, the average length of hospital stays, and health care expenditures between 1980 and 1986. Health care expenditures were adjusted to reflect Health Care

---

[1]This appendix was written by Lewin/ICF.

Financing Administration (HCFA) estimates of health expenditures by type of service and source of payment in 1986.

B. Estimation of Health Insurance Premium Payments

The public use version of the NMCUES data does not report family out-of-pocket payments for health insurance premiums. Separate procedures were used to impute premium payments. Premium payments were imputed only to NMCUES families who reported that they paid premiums for health insurance out-of-pocket.

The aged NMCUES data were matched statistically with a sample of employer health insurance plans developed by ICF Incorporated for the U.S. Small Business Administration (SBA). In this statistical matching process, each individual in the NMCUES data base who reported that he or she had health insurance coverage at his or her place of employment was assigned one of the 640 plans in the Lewin/ICF Health Plan Data Base, which is in the same firm size and industry group reported by the individual. (We also control for other plan characteristics in performing this match, including whether or not an employee contribution is required.) These plan data provide information on employer plan premiums and the amount paid by the employee. The Lewin/ICF SBA data base also includes information on health plan eligibility rules, covered services, cost sharing provisions, and employer costs.[2]

Premium payment amounts for persons with individual insurance coverage were imputed to each family in the NMCUES data based upon health insurance premium payment data reported for families in the 1977 National Medical Care Expenditures Survey (NMCES). In imputing health insurance premiums, we controlled for individual and family characteristics and whether or not dependents were covered under the plan. The family premium payment was allocated equally over all family members covered under an individual plan.

C. Actuarial Valuation of Employer Plans

Some mandatory employer health insurance proposals being discussed in Congress or by some states would require that employers provide a package of health benefits with an actuarial value which meets or exceeds a minimum actuarial value specified in the legislation. We esti-

---

[2]The sample was drawn from the Dun & Bradstreet U.S. Enterprise and Establishment Microdata file (USEEM). The sample was stratified by industry (seven groups) and firm size (five groups) to obtain estimates for these firm size and industry groups.

mated the number of persons affected by these requirements using the health plan data from the Lewin/ICF Health Plan Data Base. We estimated the actuarial value of the insurance benefits provided by each of the employer plans in the Lewin/ICF data base (described above) using an actuarial valuation model developed by Hay/Huggins Associates. We then used these actuarial values to estimate the number of persons who are in plans which provide benefits below the minimum actuarial value required under the mandatory insurance proposal. These data also permit us to estimate the number of employers affected and the increase in employer costs which would be required to bring all employer plans up to the mandated standard.

D. Utilization Response Assumptions

Although a utilization response of an increase in use of services by the newly insured is likely, it is unclear how large the response will be and what types of health care will be affected (hospital stays, physician visits, etc.). In this analysis, we assumed that among the newly insured, the level of utilization for all types of services **covered** under the new plan will increase so that on average it matches the level of utilization for persons in similar age, sex, income, and health status groups who previously had insurance.

This approach involved two major assumptions. First, we assumed that utilization for the newly insured would increase for only those services which are covered under the plan. This implicitly assumes that it is possible that the newly insured will use none of the expenditures they save on covered services to consume additional health services which are not covered under the plan. For example, if a plan excludes dental care, we did not increase utilization of dental services by the newly insured, even though it is possible that insured persons would use the money they save on covered health expenditures for additional care not covered under the plan.

A second key assumption was that health care utilization rates for the newly insured will increase to the level of the previously insured within selected age, sex, income, and health status groups. As previously uninsured individuals become insured, we assumed that their rates of utilization for each type of service will increase to the level of the previously insured in the same age, sex, income, and health status group (we controlled for a total of 67 socioeconomic groups).[3] We adjusted the following categories of health care utilization:

---

[3]The model could also use alternative assumptions on the percentage change in utilization for the newly insured derived from other sources.

- Percent with physicians' visits;
- Physicians' visits per 1,000;
- Percent with hospital stays;
- Hospital stays per 1,000;
- Hospital days per stay;
- Percent with outpatient visits;
- Outpatient visits per 1,000;
- Percent with drug expenses;
- Drug episodes per 1,000;
- Percent with emergency room visits;
- Emergency room visits per 1,000;
- Percent with other expenses; and
- Other expense episodes per 1,000.

We controlled for age, sex, income, and self-reported health status in adjusting utilization, because these are important determinants of health care utilization. Because of sample size limitations, we were unable to control for other variables, such as race and region. Also, because the sample of persons reporting themselves to be in fair or poor health was small, it was not possible to control for sex or income in those health status groups.

Appendix E

Specifications of the Illustrative Benefits Packages Used for Estimates of Commission Financing Proposal[1]

This appendix describes the covered service and cost sharing provision of the illustrative plans we selected to estimate the impacts of the Commission proposal. All individuals covered under the UNAC program were covered under the provisions of these plans except persons covered under Medicaid under current law. We assume that the UNAC program would be structured so that coverage and cost sharing for Medicaid participants would be at least as comprehensive as Medicaid under current law. The plans described in this appendix also served as the minimum benefit standard applied to the analysis of the impacts of the Commission proposal on employers and individuals with existing plans.

It is important to note that these plans were selected only for the purpose of estimates. Indeed, they are reasonable illustrations of two versions of a national package of basic services, but the Commission is not recommending a specific package. That task is left to those who would implement the Commission's proposals. Furthermore, the cost sharing provisions of these plans are slightly different from the Commission's proposals, but they are close enough for the aggregated estimates made.

---

[1]This appendix was prepared by Lewin/ICF.

A. The Basic-option Benefits Package
   1. Covered Services
      The basic-option illustrative plan would cover the following services:

      - Inpatient hospital days (no limit);
      - Inpatient physician services;
      - Outpatient hospital care under the direction of a physician, including ambulatory surgical centers;
      - Laboratory and x-ray services ordered by a physician;
      - Prenatal care;
      - Prescription drugs;
      - Psychiatric inpatient care (limit of 30 days);
      - Psychiatric outpatient care (limit of 50 visits);

      No coverage is provided for dental care.

   2. Covered Charges
      The plan would cover all charges attributed to the covered services described above up to a "reasonable and customary" amount. The reasonable and customary amount was set at the 80th percentile of charges for each type of service.

   3. Cost Sharing
      The plan would have a $100 deductible for outpatient care, including surgical and physician care, in 1988. There would be no deductible for inpatient care. The plan would reimburse 100 percent of covered charges for inpatient hospital and mental health care, 80 percent of inpatient and outpatient surgery up to the reasonable and customary amount, 80 percent of inpatient and outpatient mental health care up to the reasonable and customary amount.
      The plan also places a limit on out-of-pocket expenditures for covered services of $1,000 per person and $3,000 per family.

B. Low-option Benefits Package
   1. Covered Services
      The low-option illustrative plan would cover the following services:

      - Inpatient hospital days (up to 14 days);
      - Inpatient physician services;
      - Outpatient hospital care under the direction of a physician, including ambulatory surgical centers;

- Laboratory and x-ray services ordered by a physician;
- Prenatal care;
- Prescription drugs;
- Well-baby care;

No coverage is provided for mental health or dental care.

2. Covered Charges

The plan would cover all charges attributed to the covered services described above up to a "reasonable and customary" amount. The reasonable and customary amount was set at the 80th percentile of charges for each type of service.

3. Cost Sharing

The plan would have a $50 deductible for outpatient care, including surgical and physician care, in 1988. There would be no deductible for inpatient care. The plan would reimburse 1) 100 percent of covered charges for inpatient hospital care up to 14 days, 2) all inpatient and outpatient surgery up to the reasonable and customary amount, and 3) drug expenditures subject to a two dollar deductible per prescription. The plan does not include a limit on out-of-pocket expenditures for covered services.

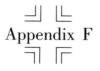

Appendix F

Methods and Data Sources

I. Service Intensity Estimates
    A. Methods

The same methods were used to estimate the potential savings for Medicare's Part A and Part B programs, and for National Health Expenditures. The process involved:

- "deflating" the budget estimates to account for population growth that inevitably affects budget size.
- "deflating" the budget estimates to account for budget growth attributable to inflation in input prices.
- calculating the difference between the projected budget and the "deflated" budget for each year; this difference is said to be the "residual" and is the portion of the budget that is attributable to rising service intensity.

    B. Data Sources

A variety of data sources were used in making the estimates. These included:

- For budget estimates:
  - Medicare Part A and Part B budgets from the Office of Management and Budget's (OMB) FY 89 mid-year estimates.
  - National Health Expenditures for hospital and physician care from the Office of the Actuary, HCFA, 1988.
- To "deflate" budgets to account for population growth:
  - OMB's Medicare mid-year enrollment estimates.
  - population estimates from HCFA's Office of the Actuary, 1988.

- To "deflate" budgets to account for price inflation:
    — Hospital Input Price Index and the Hospital Market Basket Index (for Part A and national hospital expenditures).
    — Medical Economic Index (MEI) and Physicians' Consumer Price Index (P-CPI) for physicians' services.

II. Rates of Inappropriate Use of Procedures

A. Methods

Rates of inappropriate use of procedures in the Medicare and non-Medicare populations were calculated using two different methods. For the Part B analysis, 1987 Medicare Part B claims were used for the procedures selected. For each procedure, the total allowed charges (i.e., charges actually paid) were calculated. Several of the procedures included in our list have been studied and estimates have been made as to the percent of these procedures that may be performed inappropriately (Kahn et al., 1988; Winslow et al., 1988a; Winslow et al., 1988b; Greenspan et al., 1988). This analysis assumed that these estimates are accurate and further, that all of the use said to be inappropriate would actually be eliminated. In addition, in instances where it was not possible to draw from the literature an estimate of the rate of inappropriate use, it was assumed that approximately 5 percent of a procedure's volume may be inappropriate and eliminated.

A separate analysis for the total population was performed and, where appropriate, included hospitalization costs in the analysis. Estimates were obtained from the National Center for Health Statistics of total volume performed for each procedure. These estimates are based on 1985 data; volume may well exceed the 1985 volume today, which would only boost the estimated savings. Volumes for coronary artery bypass graft (CABG) surgery and cesarean section were obtained from other sources (Medical Benefits, 1987). Hospitalization costs were not included for cataract surgery or upper gastrointestinal endoscopy, as these are most frequently performed on outpatients. Average costs were calculated for combined hospitalization and physicians' fees. For physicians' fees, Medicare's Part B file (this time assuming charges billed might be a better proxy for costs) was used. For hospitalization costs, it was assumed that Medicare charges were a good proxy for costs, and these were reduced to a per-discharge cost using a national charge-to-cost ratio.

After calculating a cost per patient procedure that captured both hospital and physician costs, inappropriate volume was estimated. It was assumed that approximately 5 percent of total volume may be reduced by the use of practice guidelines. The total number of averted procedures (i.e., 5 percent of total volume) was multiplied by the cost per procedure to obtain estimates of savings by procedure. These were summed to create a total savings figure.

B. Data Sources

The data sources for this analysis were varied. They included:

- For costs of procedures:
    - Medicare Part B allowed charges (for the Medicare analysis) and Medicare Part B billed charges (for the analysis of total population).
    - Medicare billed charges per discharge for the relevant DRG, reduced by the national charge-to-cost ratio to reflect actual costs.

- For volume estimates and rates of inappropriate use:
    - National Health Survey (NCHS, 1985).
    - Selected articles from the literature.

⌐⌐
Appendix G
⌐⌐

Comments and Dissenting Views

On as complex an issue as the health care system, the Commission never expected 100 percent support from every member. Six members have written letters with comments or dissents which are to be found in this appendix, together with the responses from the Chairmen of the Commission.

FROM THEODORE COOPER, M.D., PH.D., CHAIRMAN & CHIEF EXECUTIVE OFFICER, THE UPJOHN COMPANY

I have reviewed the final drafts of the Commission's report and accompanying materials. I am pleased that many of my strong concerns, specifically those relative to additional layers of organization and regulation, have been accommodated. I am in agreement with the statement of principles and support the thrust of the chapter on liability, although from my perspective it could be strengthened even further.

I would be less than candid, however, if I didn't express my concern over some ideas which are still prominent in the report. For example, I think that some readers might too easily and simplistically link an increasing supply of physicians with an increase in health care costs without taking into account the possibility that it could also mean improved health care. The policy implications of the link between the number of physicians and cost as expressed in the report are unclear and potentially damaging to the system itself.

I also have significant concerns over both the underlying rationale and implication of the references to unnecessary and harmful procedures. Retrospective characterizations of such procedures generally do not and cannot take into account critical determinants such as the emergency situations in which decisions must be made, the extent of information available to the medical team involved, etc. I submit that the Commission's report places too much stock in the value of retrospective studies in assessing the need for such procedures. And, in fact, the report appears to discount the link between such procedures and our concern for liability.

To my way of thinking the issues related to appropriate use of expensive procedures highlights a key deficiency in the report. As I noted earlier, I am pleased to see a reduction in recommendations for regulatory solutions; however, we do not focus attention on the importance of the role of education in improving the system.

I would also recommend a thorough revision of the "lead" paragraphs of the proposed news release; it seems to me that, in an effort to attract attention in the plethora of reports generated by the Presidential transition, the characterization of the recommendation is somewhat overstated. Not only could this diminish the credibility of the actual report, but it may also contribute to concern by constituent groups of the Commission.

In reviewing the report as well as the process which produced it, it seems to me that the greatest value should be to provoke further discussion of disparate views on approaches to achieve the vision which we have put forth. In this spirit, I think that it is essential to include comment from Commission members in a visible area of the report (i.e., not buried in the appendices).

Clearly, concerns about various facets of U.S. health programs will force themselves onto the national political agenda. This report, particularly with the inclusion of the comments of individual Commissioners, can contribute to what is bound to be an important debate.

(January 25, 1989)

FROM DOUGLAS S. PETERS, SENIOR VICE PRESIDENT, BLUE CROSS AND BLUE SHIELD ASSOCIATION

I have just received the Commission's final draft, distributed on January 27th. My intent is that these remarks be filed with the report and be "on the record."

I continue to have a number of serious concerns regarding the report's recommendations. As you know, I have expressed these concerns on many occasions—in meetings, telephone conversations and through written correspondence. I appreciate that many of my points have been recognized and are reflected in the revised materials. And yet, several of my most fundamental problems have not been adequately addressed.

I applaud and give my support to the Commission's goal of expanding access to health care. The question of how to provide health coverage for more than 37 million Americans who now lack such coverage is a matter of central concern for national health policy and for the Blue Cross and Blue Shield system. My objections are not to the stated intent of the Commission, but rather to the approach taken in the final report.

I am especially concerned about the negative impact of the proposal on the current employment-based system. In addition to providing coverage to currently uninsured individuals, the proposal also encourages movement of persons currently covered by private insurance (either employer-provided or nongroup) into the new public financing structure. Earlier drafts of the report, in fact, recognized the "substantial disincentive" for employers to continue to offer coverage directly. The report itself estimates that employers' cost associated with subsidizing the state pools would result in premiums that are about 50 percent higher than the fee (penalty) employers would pay for failing to provide coverage directly.

I also continue to be concerned about the power delegated to the state-wide boards in administering the pool and the introduction of more regulatory controls into an already heavily-regulated industry.

While I continue to have serious reservations about the final product, I can appreciate the difficulty of the task undertaken by the Commission members and staff. I look forward to participating in future discussions as these issues are considered in various forums.

(January 27, 1989)

FROM HARRY D. GARBER, VICE CHAIRMAN, THE EQUITABLE LIFE ASSURANCE SOCIETY OF THE UNITED STATES

As we have discussed on several occasions, I have serious reservations about the final work product of the Commission. While I valued the information exchange among the Commissioners and applaud much of the early analytical work done by the Commission, I have serious problems with the Commission's recommendations, which are largely unsupported by experience, analysis or research.

I request that you publish my dissenting views as part of the final report and distribute them whenever the rest of the report is distributed. In addition, there should be a reference to my dissenting views in the foreword to the Commission's report so that interested parties learn of them and know where to find them. If, for any reason, this cannot be done, I would like you to remove my name and that of my company from the Commission's report and to refrain from referencing our participation in any manner.

I regret that I have to take this position with respect to the final report, but there seems to be no way to reconcile our differences on what the Commission can and should recommend. Best wishes on your continuing quest to improve the nation's health care system.

Dissenting Views of Harry D. Garber

The Commission set noble goals for itself: to examine the problems of the American health care system and to devise recommendations to solve these problems that would be consistent with our vision of the ideal health care system.

I agree that the three inter-related problems identified by the Commission—cost, quality and access—are the key problems afflicting the nation's health care system and that the Commission's explanations of these problems are well drawn. Most of the analytical work done by the Commission's staff and the information sharing among the Commissioners in the many work sessions were extremely useful.

Unfortunately, the Commission's recommendations fall far short of this high standard of performance. Instead of being based on facts, demonstrated experience or scientific evaluation, the recommendations are characterized by partial analysis, wishful thinking and bureaucratic tendencies.

I regretfully dissent from the majority of recommendations in the report and explain my thoughts in these remarks.

Financing Access to the Health Care System. The centerpiece of the Commission's recommendations is the establishment of structure of government financed and operated health insurance pools and private insurance plans that, in combination, should assure access to the health care system for all Americans. The pools would be financed principally by an elaborate system of *new taxes* imposed on individuals and employers.

The Commission's objective is a worthy one. The difficulty that the 37 million persons without health insurance now have in accessing the health care system is a personal and national tragedy. The question is not whether it should be remedied—it must be—but when and how.

Unfortunately the Commission plan, which purports to be a comprehensive solution, is a hastily assembled structure filled with internal contradictions. We have always known that the problem of financing access to the health care system for those without insurance could be solved any time we were willing to establish a government financed and administered program and to collect sufficient taxes to support it. And in this respect the Commission plan is but another variation on an old theme.

The Commission plan, however, does not limit itself to financing access for those who presently lack such access. Instead, the Commission proposes to revamp the entire system of health care financing. There is no question that, contrary to the stated intent of the Commission to develop a plan that "builds on the American tradition of providing private health insurance through the workplace," the proposed plans will produce a significant movement of persons from employer-sponsored plans and other private insurance arrangements to the government pools. This would be the result of the Commission's proposals for a Federally-established set of minimum health care services that plans must provide, a bizarre set of mandates for handling dependent coverage, a specified employer-employee cost sharing arrangement and a rigid tax structure that ignores the immense variations in the cost of health care around the country.

Today, we have almost two-thirds of persons under age 65 covered under employer-provided health insurance arrangements and another 10% covered by other private insurance arrangements. The Commission's consultants estimate that there would be minimal shifting from employer provided coverage. But they have ignored completely the impact that using a single nationwide employer tax rate would have on employer decisions as to whether to retain private coverage or shift to pool coverage in areas with relatively high health care costs.

Before we undertake a comprehensive program to solve the access problem, particularly a program relying so heavily on tax financing and government administration, we must have confidence that the cost and quality problems are under control.

Today, the Federal and state governments, between them, administer the Medicare and Medicaid programs covering about 70 million aged, poor and disabled beneficiaries and involving annual expenditures of about $150 billion. These programs suffer from inadequate cost controls, inadequate access to care for the poor, and an inability to measure and purchase quality services for beneficiaries. Employer sponsored plans have not fared much better in cost control. If we as a nation have learned anything from our experiences with Medicaid, Medicare and from the experience of employers who "promised" retiree health benefits to employees, it is that we cannot make and expect to keep promises of future health benefits as long as the health care system remains "out of financial control." Our failure to heed this experience can lead only to disappointed citizens and increasing budgetary strains.

Even if these basic questions were not present, the Commission plan lacks some essential details. For example, the following key questions are unanswered by the report.

Who would set the tax rates and how would they be set? Who would collect the taxes? If the Federal government collects them, how would the money be distributed to the states?

What is the relationship between the tax rates, pool premiums (for employers opting to insure through the pool), and local medical costs, and how will this affect decisions by employers as to whether to offer or to retain a private health plan?

What price discounts will the pool be able to obtain from providers? What cost shifting to private payers will result?

How many jobs will be lost as a result of these additional employer costs? Is the assertion in the report that less than 100,000 jobs will be lost reasonable in light of the additional employer tax/benefit plan expenses?

Cost and Quality. The Commission fails to address substantially the question of the rising cost of the nation's health care system. The central recommendation in this respect is that the state agency administering the pool take on the major responsibility for achieving overall health care cost control within the state and that private payers be permitted to benefit from any negotiated price structures.

There are at least two major problems with this proposal, both of which are likely and either of which would render it ineffective. These are:

- The primary task of the state agency must be, in the end, to keep expenses less than or equal to revenue. If the history of Medicaid is any guide, this will result in very low reimbursement rates to those who provide services to the pool beneficiaries, with the resultant cost shifting to private payers. Attempting to represent all payers would present an unresolvable conflict of interest to the state agencies.

- The American system of government involves built-in separations of power among the several branches of government and between Federal and local authorities. It requires, as a consequence, detailed legislation in matters affecting the rights of its citizens. I cannot conceive of a state entity having the legislative authority and expert skills to make the business decisions and judgements required to achieve the necessary cost/quality results. In no other sector of our society have we turned to a governmentally run system as a cure all for problems. Indeed, the history of our government's administration of the current Medicare and Medicaid programs gives no comfort that it would be equal to the challenge presented by the Commission.

With respect to the issue of quality, the Commission recommends a national quality improvement initiative, a major component of which would be sharply increased funding of research on the results of clinical practice. This research would provide a basis for professional standards of practice. There is no question that such research is needed, that substantial additional resources will be required to fund it, and that the professional societies must be involved in the development and implementation of the necessary professional standards. The substantial question that remains is whether the levying of a $500 million tax is the most effective way to approach the funding of this work, particularly given the current short supply of experienced and interested researchers in this area. I do not believe it is.

Suggestions for Action. Our health care system is unique in the world. I believe that it is possible to preserve its unique qualities while remedying the existing problems of cost, quality and lack of access. But it requires an immense social and economic engineering project involving providers, payers, governments, patients, insurers and other intermediaries, unions, and other interested parties. In the end the providers must be organized to provide quality and cost-effective services, and buyers of their services must possess sufficient market power to assure that this is the case. And all of this must be done locality by locality, because the health care system is composed of hundreds of local markets.

What we need to recognize is that this result can happen only if someone makes it happen and the only "somebodies" that can make it happen today are the employers, working with their insurers. The major employers, who pay most of the bills presently, must recognize that they are the only entities with the resources and incentives to solve the cost/quality problems and that they need to undertake the hard work of doing so. Instead of recommending a government program that purports to solve the cost/quality problem for the employers—if it works—the Commission should have taken the more realistic route of challenging the employer community to assume the initiative and a major share of the responsibility for the solution of these cost and quality problems.

Conclusion. The Commission report is worthy of review more for its definition of current problems in the health care system and its vision of the future than for its detailed recommendations. The recommendations will not help us to achieve our vision. The report is, indeed, a missed

opportunity to have a positive impact on the health care delivery
system.

(January 24, 1989)

RESPONSE TO HARRY D. GARBER FROM THE COMMISSION CHAIRMEN

We are in receipt of your letter of January 24, 1989. You and Equitable
have been strong supporters of our effort from the very beginning and
have given generously of your time and resources, and for this we are
grateful.

We are particularly pleased you agree with the Commission's diagnosis and analysis of the key interrelated problems of cost, quality and
access. This is important since it is clear that unless we understand and
agree on the nature of the problems it is unlikely we will solve them.

Your disagreements relate to a number of the Commission's proposed solutions and here we must take sharp issue with a number of
your conclusions. You suggest that the Commission has failed to "address substantially" the issue of rising costs, you question our approach
to the quality problem, and conclude that employers and their insurers
are the only entities with the resources and incentives to solve the cost
and quality problems.

We note your concern of a possible adverse effect on the insurance
industry. Our proposals serve the public interest, and not at the expense
or benefit of any one group. We do feel that there will continue to be an
important role for the insurance industry.

We have learned over the past two and one-half years that no single
group in America, including the federal government, can alone solve the
problems of cost, quality, and access. It also seems increasingly clear that
no single company feels the problems can be solved without new
strategies.

This is why from the very beginning we agreed that only a comprehensive, systemic strategy could succeed and why we call for a pub-
lic/private partnership. We strongly rejected a totally governmental
solution.

We feel the cost problem cannot be separated from the quality and
access problems. Until we can better define quality and appropriateness
we cannot know what is worth providing access to or what is worth
paying for. That is why a key element of our strategy involves the development of guidelines for quality and appropriateness. Our quality initiative is a building block on which an effective cost containment strategy

can be built. Our proposal will also make costs explicit and address the cost shifting which now effectively frustrates cost containment efforts.

Thank you for the many ways in which you have contributed to the Commission's work.

(January 29, 1989)

FROM WALTON E. BURDICK, VICE PRESIDENT OF PERSONNEL, I.B.M.

I have been thinking a great deal about the task the Commission has labored over for the past two years. Having worked diligently to take into account all of the various points of view and the interests of multiple segments of our society, it is no wonder we have found the deliberations to be so difficult, particularly at the concluding stages. While commissions of this sort frequently face these kinds of problems, the issues on our agenda have resisted solutions for so long, our dilemma is even greater.

While I believe most Commissioners agree in general with the vision that has been drafted, consensus on other specific proposals continues to be a problem. In my own case, I remain troubled by the following:

1. The report contains no real solutions to the cost escalation problem facing us today.

2. Access as the dominant theme, which will add significant cost to the system and create demand, without balance on the cost containment side, is unacceptable.

3. Solving a societal problem with an employer solution (employers paying by providing benefits or paying the required tax) is unhealthy for our economy, anticompetitive and unfair to private business.

4. The variety of mandates, including a federally designed package of required benefits, the possibility of states superceding that package with an even richer package mandated within states, and a new threshold defining who must be considered an employee, are all onerous. These kinds of decisions should be determined within the employer/employee relationship.

Unless these issues are resolved in a manner satisfactory for my company and business in general, then I too will fall in the category of those dissenting from the final package.

(January 9, 1989)

RESPONSE TO WALTON E. BURDICK FROM THE COMMISSION CHAIRMEN

We are in receipt of your letter of January 9, 1989, noting your concerns in a number of areas. We will publish your letter as part of our final report.

As noted in discussions with you and your staff, we do feel our proposal contains a strong cost containment strategy and that access, though important, is not the dominant element of our strategy, but rather one of three major issues to be addressed. In fact, all three elements of cost, quality and access are equally important and must be addressed together since they are so interrelated.

We share your concerns that whatever solution this nation finally adopts must not be unhealthy for our economy, not be anti-competitive, and not unfair to private business. We have made these points forcefully in the final report. You note concern with the funding mechanism proposed. Our report notes that funding for our access proposal could also come from general revenues.

In the meantime, we are grateful for IBM's support and extensive involvement with staff and resources over these past two years and especially for the support you and Jack Rogers have given personally.

(January 29, 1989)

FROM J. BRUCE JOHNSTON, J.D., EXECUTIVE VICE PRESIDENT, USX

I have reviewed, painstakingly, the January, 1989 draft of the Commission's report "For the Health of a Nation."

I conclude, with genuine regret, but little uncertainty, that USX could never support these proposals or anything like them. My disagreement with the proposals is so profound that I am obliged to request that this letter of dissent be published and distributed with the Report *or* that my name and the name of USX Corporation be removed from the report and the letterhead of the Commission before any press release or other distribution could be interpreted as tacit assent by USX, or me, to these proposals. We take this action with personal regret, but we could not be associated with proposals that are so contrary to all the experience which forms our view that market forces, individual responsibility, government as provider of last resort, and the linkage of public accountability in the political process via revenue raising to finance the promised benefits, represents the best prospect and the most responsible course for providing optimal health care delivery.

From the inception of this project, I advised in the plainest imaginable terms that there was little likelihood that the combination of adverse parties (buyers and sellers) included in the composition of this Commission could ever produce a report that each could support.

We agree that medical care in this country has far-reaching, and deep-seated problems in need of solution. The problems are presented extensively in the report and we generally concur with those descriptions. But diagnosis is the easier part of this problem. Anyone might accept the broad generalities presented in the "Vision" Statement, but even they short-change the *sine-qua-non* issue of cost containment. This Report's fundamental failure to deal hard-headedly with cost containment fatally flaws its remaining wish-list. Cost containment is dismissed as an afterthought rather than recognized as the core issue. Where else but the health care industry could its providers be so ambitious about selling more and more product with less care about how it will all be paid for?

Here are some specific objections.

- The proposed system would expansively increase access by just majestically proposing to insure everyone! But the Report contains *no* offsetting, concrete, identifiable, time-tested, financing controls to keep aggregate medical cost from its currently reeling consumption of more and more of our gross national product. Even the weakly conceived cost containment references mentioned in the Report are extended so far into the future and are so gossamer in nature as to render the entire proposal frivolous.

  While health care costs soar above inflation, this Report sees the solution as more "access." The proposed remedy is not new at all—its prescription for cost containment is unbelievable—it proposes to throw more money at the problem—up front, and to then somehow hope for cost reduction on the other side of the rainbow. If our medical industry has proved anything—surely it is that this industry can spend money without limit, and the more money we want to feed it, the more the industry will grow to first expect it, and then to demand it, as a societal entitlement.

- The proposed scheme would *mandate* a government specified complement of benefits for every single individual person in this country, but that's not all—it then proposes, contemporaneously, to remove from elected officials all responsibility and all political accountability for collecting the revenue to pay for the increased availability of benefits. It would be a mistake of the most fundamental and far-reaching significance to break the linkage between publicly promising legislative benefits and being publicly accountable for raising the money to pay for them.

Even though these proposals argue that an insurance base represents some kind of individual responsibility, they ignore the reality that employers would pay most of the bill *and* that they would now have to carry, in their product prices, the cost of expanded medical benefits for everyone imaginable. All this while manufacturers fight for competitive survival in world markets, and while our politicians simultaneously ladle out more and more parallel entitlements with their attendant transfer costs, all of which have contributed heavily to our awesome federal deficit. This proposal not only fails to ameliorate each of these phenomena—it is a formulation for making each of them worse.

- Another area where we just as plainly are repelled by the proposal is the idea that each State now be authorized to add an additional layer of Health Benefits for all the pooled participants in its own jurisdiction. Be assured that all the States would soon set the benefit levels of private employers by determining politically whether or not a newly proposed X_1 tax would be charged to covered employers. That clearly places any covered business in double jeopardy, and is obviously a mandating of benefits in thinly disguised form.

  The ERISA preemption is the only current protection which employers have against the ravenous appetite of State politicians for more and more mandated benefits. We would, of course, oppose any attempt to remove that preemption, and cannot imagine any employer of consequence, after analysis, not finding that same conclusion ineluctable! (The only basis for a different conclusion, which we can conceive of, is the possibility that a large private employer might wish to cost-shift its own medical expenses from shareholders to taxpayers by supporting a national health insurance program which leads to federally guaranteed health benefits for everybody. That will, in turn, pump vastly more private and public money into health care on an absolute basis, but it might reduce the employment cost of a large individual employer on a relative basis.)

  We do not believe that such a development would be good for our society, for prospects of coping with the federal deficit, or that it represents a wise consumption of limited medical resources. Those who consume any product but get no share in the cost of its consumption and get no responsibility for allocating their own consumer dollars, and assume none of the responsibility for the consequent misallocation of resources this proposal will produce, will soon generate mind-boggling consequences for American taxpayers. When the government backs all the bets, irresponsible betting soon follows. The FSLIC fiasco will pale by comparison to the subsidy nightmare which would evolve from a scheme like this one.

- Significant cost-shifting in current health care arrangements results plainly from the present refusal of Medicaid to pay the direct cost of the very benefits it guarantees. This proposal would expand the group receiving government mandated health care benefits all of which are to be purchased through negotiation with existing State Agencies. Consequently, the States (whose policies are always formulated politically) will use this increased purchasing power to dictate even lower payments to its providers, thereby fostering crushing cost-shifting to private employers who are expected to purchase similar benefits for their employees. But employers will be prevented from placing their own employees in the "pool" (which they will nevertheless be taxed to pay for) if they compensate their own employees well (250% of poverty level). Even if an employer gets an option to elect the State Agencies' medical prices, few, if any, private employers would have the market power to force their providers to sell medical services at these same prices. The largest private corporation pales by comparison with the purchasing power of the Federal Government thru Medicaid, Medicare, or other sovereignties.

- The report speaks only generally (and perhaps even too broadly) of quality "weaknesses" in current medical services. The report, however, asks boldly for more money for research, it proposes "A New Unifying Quality Improvement Initiative" and it spells out the need for a national data base. But, there are *no* clearly defined proposals for measuring quality, there are *no* clearly defined proposals for improving quality and there are *no* suggested methods for license suspension of physicians selling poor quality medicine. In plain English, no tangible quality improvement mechanism whatsoever!

  What else can come from the composition of such a group? Congress exempts itself from all the regulatory statutes it mandates for everyone else, and health care providers, with the same self-interest as any other group, proposes the same kind of scheme—what the medical providers want is defined in firm dollars, precise time tables, and clear mandates—what is required of them is limited to an acknowledgment of the problem, and a lot of hope.

No one quarrels with the weaknesses in our present health care. But the first tenet of both medical and legal education is the maxim to: 'First Do No Harm'! These proposals under the guise of addressing the cost fire, call for more financial fuel. It would be bad enough not to help—but these proposals would harm. If health care *costs* are not brought under control, health care outcomes will worsen.

The proposals offered by this Commission emphasize more access (which advantages providers and increases cost), they emphasize more research (which advantages providers and increases cost), they emphasize more education (which advantages providers and increases cost), and solutions for the malpractice problem (which advantages providers).

Under these proposals, health care delivery would be given a substantial infusion of still more money, but absolutely nothing is demanded or required from those who will consume these new benefits, and nothing is offered to protect or limit the liability of those who must pay for them.

We will be obliged to oppose these proposals, as forcefully as we can.

(January 23, 1989)

RESPONSE TO J. BRUCE JOHNSTON FROM THE COMMISSION CHAIRMEN

We are in receipt of your letter of January 23, 1989, noting your dissent. We will publish it along with our final report. A number of your concerns were similar to those of Messrs. Garber and Burdick and we enclose our replies to them for your information.

The Commission designed a cost control strategy that we feel will work over time. It is clear you do not agree. We welcome your suggestions as to how this nation can control costs, assure quality, and provide Americans with equitable access to needed services.

We wish you had been able to participate in at least some of the Commission's meetings, because a number of Commissioners started out with the position you now hold, but after hearing the extensive testimony the Commission invited, and joining in Commission dialogue, their views changed.

(January 29, 1989)

FROM JAMES H. SAMMONS, M.D., EXECUTIVE VICE PRESIDENT, AMERICAN MEDICAL ASSOCIATION

I appreciate the additional time for us and other members of the Commission to do a thorough review of the National Leadership Commission's final report. At my request, the AMA staff has conducted a detailed analysis of the report. We have many serious objections in the philosophy it represents and in specific solutions proposed.

1. The plan calls for total restructuring of the health care system to central control and heavy regulation which is essentially a national health insurance scheme. There is no evidence that such a system is more cost effective and, in fact, under this proposal would create major new government programs at considerable expense.

2. The Commission itself estimates the draft plan would cost employers and workers $71 billion.

3. A number of organizations are aggressively pursuing new quality assurance initiatives. There is no evidence to support any benefit from a national coordinating quality assurance board. This proposal alone is estimated to cost $500 million raised through a payroll tax and more importantly removes from hospitals and physicians the primary responsibility to assure quality of care. Furthermore, the report assumes a much more independent capability to define, quantify and measure quality and efficiency than currently exists ignoring the profession which has better expertise.

4. The report fails to address the long term care issue which may be the most difficult and costly one facing health care.

5. Dismantling the Medicaid Agencies only to create new State Boards whose purpose is ill conceived and poorly defined is wasteful and unnecessary.

Imposition of a completely untested new system is not, in our view, politically or economically practical nor does it do much to solve the real problems at hand. Our efforts would be better directed to specific and well designed reforms that address identified problems in the system. For example:

1. The Health Policy Agenda Subcommittee on Medicaid will make public in February a detailed plan to substantially reform and expand the Medicaid program.

2. The AMA has proposed in legislation form an extensive plan for Medicare reforms including detailed cost analyses by expert actuaries.

3. The AMA will collaborate with the Rand Corporation on a major quality assurance initiative to establish practice parameters for quality assurance reviews.

4. The AMA will continue to work with HCFA, PPRC and others on specific physician payment reform proposals such as RBRVS.

This is not to imply that AMA's initiatives are the only ones. But we believe real life, evolutionary and practical solutions such as these are the best approach to the current problems we all recognize and constructively look to resolve.

In addition to our objections with the content of this report, I continue to be dissatisfied with the process that has produced it. I do not believe the full membership of the Commission was adequately represented at the table during these discussions and I do not believe the final report represents a consensus of their views. The report is negative to medicine and physicians and editorializes in an unacceptable manner throughout. I use as comparison the Health Policy Agenda which was truly broad based and which established a rational process for reaching consensus with 195 organizations representing business, consumers, insurors, government and others over a five year period.

I have considered at great length constructive recommendations we could make to improve the report. Unfortunately, however, the tone, the philosophy and the solutions are so unacceptable throughout that I see no way in which I personally, or the AMA as an organization, could support the report.

(December 15, 1988)

* * *

I cannot, nor can the American Medical Association, support the final report of the National Leadership Commission on Health Care. This action is taken after our recent thorough review and analysis of the proposed final report of the Commission.

We share agreement with some of the broad principles set out in the report, including the fundamental principle of universal access. However, I find that the program which is contained in the final report does not carry forward the principles in a manner which would be in the best interests of our citizens.

In my December 15, 1988 letter to you regarding the Commission's draft report, I stated our serious objections to the report's direction of essentially restructuring the entire health care system toward a system of central control and heavy government regulation. That direction has not changed in the final version. Likewise, the tone of the report remains unduly negative to medicine and physicians and editorializes in an unacceptable manner. For example, we find it totally unacceptable to cite in the conclusion to Chapter One, and thus to infer acquiescence by the Commission, a quotation stating that ". . . much of the medical care in this country is unnecessary, is of no demonstrated value to those who receive it, and some of it is harmful."

As also stated in our December 15th letter, we remain dissatisfied with the process by which the report was produced. In my opinion the full membership of the Commission was not adequately represented during meetings. Consequently, I must question whether the proposed final draft represents a consensus of Commission opinion.

It is true that there are problems and shortcomings in our health care system. It is equally true that our country is acknowledged as having the finest health care available in the world today. The ultimate goal should be to seek necessary improvements while preserving the full benefits of our system enjoyed by so many. This is the goal of the AMA, namely, to provide increased access to a system providing the best health care possible. We will, therefore, continue to advocate our policy of expanded eligibility and coverage under Medicaid to all persons below poverty, creation of state risk pools with voucher assistance as necessary for the uninsured above poverty, and for fundamental financing reform of the Medicare program to assure continued health care for the elderly. In addition, we will continue to promote constructive measures to enhance the quality of care.

I respectfully request that any dissenting views of Commissioners be acknowledged early in the report. I also request that this letter and my letter of December 15, 1988, showing my disagreement with the report, be included as an appendix to the report. If the letters are not to be so published, then remove my name as a Commissioner.

(January 24, 1989)

RESPONSE TO JAMES H. SAMMONS FROM THE COMMISSION CHAIRMEN

We are in receipt of your letters of December 15, 1988 and January 24, 1989. They will be published as part of our final report.

We are pleased you recognize and agree that problems exist in the areas of cost, quality, and access and that you support fundamental financing reforms, universal access, state risk pools, and the aggressive pursuit of quality assurance initiatives. These are major elements of the series of comprehensive reforms we propose. As you know, we rejected piecemeal solutions because we felt that approach has failed.

At the same time, you make a number of allegations with which we must in good conscience take issue. During the two-and-one-half years of Commission deliberations, the Commission never supported heavy regulation or strong central control. In fact, the Commission specifically rejected a totally governmental solution. That is why our strategy builds so extensively on elements of the existing system, includes attempts to improve the market, and why it calls for a new public/private partnership with involvement of physicians and other health professionals, especially in the area of quality assurance.

In addition, we believe thoughtful physicians will be strongly supportive of the Commission, agreeing with the principles of universal access, fair compensation of providers, restoration of clinical freedom to providers, and our strong emphasis on the need to do all possible to enhance the doctor-patient relationship.

From its inception there was intense involvement of Commissioners in the process and a desire to serve the public interest, thereby solving the problems instead of assigning blame. We believe a fair reading of the report would show that the members succeeded in that aim.

We appreciate what time you were able to give this effort and welcome any opportunity to work with you toward our mutual goal of improving and strengthening our health care system.

(February 6, 1989)

Bibliography

ARTICLES

Journal or Magazine Articles

Alper, P., "Medical Practice in the Competitive Market," *NEJM* 316(6):337–339, February 5, 1987.

Altman, S., and Rodwin, M., "Halfway Competitive Markets and Ineffective Regulation: The American Health Care System," *Journal of Health Politics, Policy and Law* 13(2):323–339, Summer 1988.

American Medical Association, "Board of Trustees Report: Report of the Special Task Force on Professional Liability and Insurance and the Advisory Panel on Professional Liability," *JAMA* 257(6):810–812, February 13, 1987.

Anderson, G., and Erickson, J., "National Medical Spending," *Health Affairs* 6(3):96–104, Fall 1987.

Angell, M., "Cost Containment and the Physician," *JAMA* 254(9):1203–1207, September 6, 1985.

Ansell, D., and Schiff, R., "Patient Dumping: Status, Implications, and Policy Recommendations," *JAMA* 257(11):1500–1502, March 20, 1987.

Antman, K., Schnipper, L., and Frei III, E., "The Crisis in Clinical Cancer Research: Third-Party Insurance and Investigational Therapy," *NEJM* 319(1):46–48, July 7, 1988.

Bailar, J., and Smith, E., "Progress Against Cancer?" *NEJM* 314(19):1226–1232, May 8, 1986.

Barer, M., Evans, R., and Labelle, R., "Fee Controls as Cost Control: Tales from the Frozen North," *Milbank Quarterly* 66(1):1–64, 1988.

Barry, M., Mulley, A., et al., "Watchful Waiting vs. Immediate Transurethral Resection for Symptomatic Prostatism," *JAMA* 259(20):3010–3017, May 27, 1988.

Berrien, R., "What Future for Primary Care Private Practice?" *NEJM* 316(6):334–337, February 5, 1987.

Blendon, R., "The Public's View of the Future of Health Care," *JAMA* 259(24):3587–3593, June 24, 1988.

Blendon, R., "Three Systems: A Comparative Survey," *Health Management Quarterly* 11(1):2–10, First Quarter 1989.

Blendon, R., "What Should Be Done About the Uninsured Poor?" *JAMA* 260(21):3176–3177, December 2, 1988.

Blendon, R., et al., "Uncompensated Care by Hospitals or Public Insurance for the Poor: Does It Make a Difference?" *NEJM* 314(18):1160–1163, May 1, 1986.

Block, J., Regenstreif, D., and Griner, P., "A Community Hospital Payment Experiment Outperforms National Experience: The Hospital Experimental Payment Program in Rochester, NY," *JAMA* 257(2):193–197, January 9, 1987.

Bock, R., "The Pressure to Keep Prices High at a Walk-in Clinic," *NEJM* 319(12):785–787, September 22, 1988.

Bovbjerg, R., "Insuring the Uninsured Through Private Action: Ideas and Initiatives," *Inquiry* 23:403–418, Winter 1986.

Bovbjerg, R., and Koller, C., "State Health Insurance Pools: Current Performance, Future Prospects," *Inquiry* 23:111–121, Summer 1986.

Brook, R., and Kosecoff, J., "Competition and Quality," *Health Affairs* 7(3):150–161, Summer 1988.

Brook, R., and Lohr, K., "Efficacy, Effectiveness, Variations, and Quality," *Medical Care* 23(5):710–722, May 1985.

Brook, R., Lohr, K., et al., "Geographic Variations in the Use of Services: Do They Have Any Clinical Significance?" *Health Affairs* 3(2):63–73, Summer 1984.

Bucci, V., and Reiss, J., "Technology Assessment of Medical Devices Under Medicare: Who Should Examine 'Safety and Effectiveness'?" *Food Drug Cosmetic Law Journal* 40(4):445–455, October 1985.

Bucci, V., Reiss, J., and Hall, N., "New Obstacles in the Path of Marketing New Medical Devices," *Journal of Health Care Technology* 2(2):81–96, Fall 1985.

Bulger, R., "Archie Cochrane Revisited," *JAMA* 260(9):1284, September 2, 1988.

Burda, D., "Liability Reshapes Hospital/Physician Relationships," *Hospitals*, pp. 56–60, April 5, 1987.

Callahan, D., "Adequate Health Care and an Aging Society: Are They Morally Compatible?" *Daedalus*, pp. 247–267, Winter 1986.

Callahan, D., "Allocating Health Resources," *Center Report*, April/May 1988, p. 18.

Caper, P., "Solving the Medical Care Dilemma," *NEJM* 318(23):1535–1536, June 9, 1988.

Caper, P., "Variations in Medical Practice: Implications for Health Policy," *Health Affairs* 3(2):110–119, Summer 1984.

"The Cesarean Future," *Medical Benefits*, October 31, 1987.

Chambers, B., and Norris, J., "Outcome in Patients with Asymptomatic Neck Bruits," *NEJM* 315(14):860–865, October 2, 1986.

Chassin, M., Brook, R., et al., "Variations in the Use of Medical and Surgical Services by the Medicare Population," *NEJM* 314(5):285–290, January 30, 1986.

Chassin, M., Kosecoff, J., et al., "Does Inappropriate Use Explain Geographic Variations in the Use of Health Care Services?" *JAMA* 258(18):2533–2537, November 13, 1987.

Chassin, M., Kosecoff, J., et al., "How Coronary Angiography Is Used," *JAMA* 258(18):2543–2545, November 13, 1987.

Couch, N., Tilney, N., et al., "The High Cost of Low-Frequency Events: The Anatomy and Economics of Surgical Mishaps," *NEJM* 304(11):634–637, March 12, 1981.

Culliton, B., "Integrity of Research Papers Questioned: Two Researchers from NIH Allege That the Scientific Literature May Be Full of Minor Errors; Others Argue They Have Very Little Evidence," *Science* 235:422–423, January 23, 1987.

Curran, W., "Medical Peer Review of Physician Competence and Performance:

Legal Immunity and the Antitrust Laws," *NEJM* 316(10):597–598, March 5, 1987.

Danzon, P., "The Frequency and Severity of Medical Malpractice Claims: New Evidence," *Law and Contemporary Problems* 49(2):57–84, Spring 1986.

de Lissovoy, G., "Medicare and Heart Transplants: Will Lightning Strike Twice?" *Health Affairs* 7(4):61–71, Fall 1988.

Donabedian, A., "The Quality of Care: How Can It Be Assessed?" *JAMA* 260(12):1743–1748, September 23/30, 1988.

Dubovsky, S., "Coping with Entitlement in Medical Education," *NEJM* 315(26):1672–1674, December 25, 1986.

Dundes, L., "The Evolution of Maternal Birthing Position," *American Journal of Public Health* 77(5):636–641, May 1987.

Eddy, D., "Variations in Physician Practice: The Role of Uncertainty," *Health Affairs* 3(2):74–89, Summer 1984.

Eddy, D., Hasselblad, V., et al., "The Value of Mammography Screening in Women Under Age 50 Years," *JAMA* 259(10):1512–1519, March 11, 1988.

Egdahl, R., "Ways for Surgeons to Increase the Efficiency of Their Use of Hospitals," *NEJM* 309(19):1184–1187, November 10, 1983.

Ellwood, P., "Shattuck Lecture—Outcomes Management: A Technology of Patient Experience," *NEJM* 318(23):1549–1556, June 9, 1988.

Enthoven, A., "Managed Competition: An Agenda for Action," *Health Affairs* 7(3):25–47, Summer 1988.

Enthoven, A., "A New Proposal to Reform the Tax Treatment of Health Insurance," *Health Affairs* 3(1):21–39, Spring 1984.

Epstein, A., Begg, C., and McNeil, B., "The Use of Ambulatory Testing in Prepaid and Fee-for-Service Group Practices: Relation to Perceived Profitability," *NEJM* 314(17):1089–1094, April 24, 1986.

Faltermay, E., "Medical Care's Next Revolution," *Fortune*, pp. 126–133, October 10, 1988.

Feinstein, A., "An Additional Basic Science for Clinical Medicine: I. The Constraining Fundamental Paradigms," *Annals of Internal Medicine* 99(3):393–397, September 1983.

Feinstein, A., "An Additional Basic Science for Clinical Medicine: II. The Limitations of Randomized Trials," *Annals of Internal Medicine* 99(4):544–550, October 1983.

Feinstein, A., "An Additional Basic Science for Clinical Medicine: III. The Challenges of Comparison and Measurement," *Annals of Internal Medicine* 99(5):705–712, November 1983.

Feinstein, A., "An Additional Basic Science for Clinical Medicine: IV. The Development of Clinimetrics," *Annals of Internal Medicine* 99(6):843–848, December 1983.

Feinstein, A., "The Intellectual Crisis in Clinical Science: Medaled Models and Muddled Mettle," *Perspectives in Biology and Medicine* 30(2):215–230, Winter 1987.

Feinstein, A., and Horwitz, R., "Double Standards, Scientific Methods, and Epidemiologic Research," *NEJM* 307:1611–1617, December 23, 1982.

Feinstein, A., Sosin, D., and Wells, C., "The Will Rogers Phenomenon: Stage Migration and New Diagnostic Techniques as a Source of Misleading Statistics for Survival in Cancer," *NEJM* 312(25):1604–1608, June 20, 1985.

Feldman, R., and Sloan, F., "Competition Among Physicians, Revisited," *Journal of Health Politics, Policy and Law* 13(2):239–261, Summer 1988.

Feldstein, P., Wickizer, T., and Wheeler, J., "Private Cost Containment: The Effects of Utilization Review Programs on Health Care Use and Expenditures," *NEJM* 318(20):1310–1314, May 19, 1988.

Fowler, F., Wennberg, J., et al., "Symptom Status and Quality of Life Following Prostatectomy," *JAMA* 259(20):3018–3022, May 27, 1988.

Fowles, J., Bunker, J., and Schurman, D., "Hip Surgery Data Yield Quality Indicators," *Business and Health* 4(8):44–46, June 1987.

Fuchs, V., "The 'Competition Revolution' in Health Care," *Health Affairs* 7(3):5–24, Summer 1988.

Fujii, M., and Reich, M., "Rising Medical Costs and the Reform of Japan's Health Insurance System," *Health Policy* 9:9–24, 1988.

Gabel, J., Jajich-Toth, C., et al., "The Changing World of Group Health Insurance," *Health Affairs* 7(3):48–65, Summer 1988.

Ginzberg, E., "Cost Containment—Imaginary and Real," *NEJM* 308(20):1220–1224, May 19, 1983.

Ginzberg, E., "For-Profit Medicine: A Reassessment," *NEJM* 319(12):757–760, September 22, 1988.

Goldman, L., "Diagnostic Advances vs. the Value of the Autopsy: 1912–1980," *Archives of Pathology and Laboratory Medicine* 108:501–505, June 1984.

Goldman, L., and Cook, E., "The Decline in Ischemic Heart Disease Mortality Rates: An Analysis of the Comparative Effects of Medical Interventions and Changes in Lifestyle," *Annals of Internal Medicine* 101:825–836, December 1984.

Gosfield, A., "Navigating Through JCAH's New Quality Assurance and Medical Staff Standards," *HealthSpan* 4(2):3–9, February 1987.

Graboys, T., Headley, A., et al., "Results of a Second-Opinion Program for Coronary Artery Bypass Graft Surgery," *JAMA* 258(12):1611–1614, September 25, 1987.

Greenberg, W., "Introduction," *Journal of Health Politics, Policy and Law* 13(2):223–225, Summer 1988.

Greenfield, S., Aronow, H., et al., "Flaws in Mortality Data: The Hazards of Ignoring Comorbid Disease," *JAMA* 260(15):2253–2255, October 21, 1988.

Greenspan, A., Kay, H., et al., "Incidence of Unwarranted Implantation of Permanent Cardiac Pacemakers in a Large Medical Population," *NEJM* 318(3):158–163, January 21, 1988.

Greer, A., "The State of the Art Versus the State of the Science: The Diffusion of New Medical Technologies into Practice," *International Journal of Technology Assessment in Health Care* 4(1):5–26, 1988.

Griner, P., and Glaser, R., "Misuse of Laboratory Tests and Diagnostic Procedures," *NEJM* 307(21):1336–1339, November 18, 1982.

Hartley, R., Charlton, J., et al., "Patterns of Physicians' Use of Medical Resources in Ambulatory Settings," *American Journal of Public Health* 77(5):565–567, May 1987.

Harvey, M., and Levine, R., "The Risk of Research Procedures: Methodologic Problems and Proposed Standards," *Clinical Research* 31(2):126–139, April 1983.

Heilman, R., "What's Wrong with Radiology," *NEJM* 306(8):477–479, February 25, 1982.

Held, P., Pauly, M., and Diamond, L., "Survival Analysis of Patients Undergoing Dialysis," *JAMA* 257(5):645–650, February 6, 1987.

Hewitt Associates, "Salaried Employee Benefits Provided by Major U.S. Employers in 1986," *Medical Benefits*, June 15, 1987.

Himmelstein, D., and Woolhandler, S., "Cost Without Benefit: Administrative Waste in U.S. Health Care," *NEJM* 314(7):441–445, February 13, 1986.

Hsiao, W., Braun, P., et al., "Estimating Physicians' Work for a Resource-Based Relative-Value Scale," *NEJM* 319(13):835–841, September 29, 1988.

Hsiao, W., Braun, P., et al., "Results and Policy Implications of the Resource-Based Relative-Value Study," *NEJM* 319(13):881–888, September 29, 1988.

Hsiao, W., Braun, P., et al., "Results, Potential Effects, and Implementation Issues of the Resource-Based Relative-Value Scale," *JAMA* 260(16):2429–2438, October 28, 1988.

Hubbard, S., Henney, J., and DeVita, V., "A Computer Data Base for Information on Cancer Treatment," *NEJM* 316(6):315–318, February 5, 1987.

Hubbell, F., Greenfield, S., et al., "The Impact of Routine Admission Chest X-Ray Films on Patient Care," *NEJM* 312(4):209–213, January 24, 1985.

Iglehart, J., "Health Policy Report: Japan's Medical Care System," *NEJM* 319(12):807–812, September 22, 1988.

Jacobs, B., and Weissert, W., "Using Home Equity to Finance Long-Term Care," *Journal of Health Politics, Policy and Law* 12(1):77–95, Spring 1987.

Jacobson, K., Branch, L., and Nelson, H., "Laboratory Tests in Chronic Urticaria," *JAMA* 243(16):1644–1646, April 25, 1980.

Jacobson, P., and Rosenquist, C., "The Introduction of Low-Osmolar Contrast Agents in Radiology: Medical, Economic, Legal, and Public Policy Issues," *JAMA* 260(11):1586–1592, September 16, 1988.

James, T., "Cascades, Collusions, and Conflicts in Cardiology," *JAMA* 259(16):2454–2455, April 22/29, 1988.

Jencks, S., and Kay, T., "Do Frail, Disabled, Poor, and Very Old Medicare Beneficiaries Have Higher Hospital Charges?" *JAMA* 257(2):198–202, January 9, 1987.

Jencks, S., Williams, D., and Kay, T., "Assessing Hospital-Associated Deaths from Discharge Data: The Role of Length of Stay and Comorbidities," *JAMA* 260(15):2240–2246, October 21, 1988.

Jennett, B., "Assessment of Clinical Technologies: Importance for Provision and Use," *International Journal of Technology Assessment in Health Care* 4(3):435–445, 1988.

Jennett, B., "High Technology Medicine and Quality of Life," *International Journal of Technology Assessment in Health Care* 3(1):51–60, 1987.

Joe, T., Meltzer, J., and Yu, P., "Arbitrary Access to Care: The Case for Reforming Medicaid," *Health Affairs* 4(1):59–74, Spring 1985.

Johns, L., "Selective Contracting in California," *Health Affairs* 4(3):32–48, Fall 1985.

Johns, L., and Jones, M., "Physician Response to Selective Contracting in California," *Health Affairs* 6(4):59–69, Winter 1987.

Justice, D., "State Initiatives in Reforming Long-Term Care," *Business and Health* 4(2):14–19, December 1986.

Kahn, K., Kosecoff, J., et al., "The Use and Misuse of Upper Gastrointestinal Endoscopy," *Annals of Internal Medicine* 109:664–670, 1988.

Kane, R., and Kane, R., "The Feasibility of Universal Long-Term-Care Benefits: Ideas from Canada," *NEJM* 312(21):1357–1364, May 23, 1985.

Kaplan, E., Sheiner, L., et al., "The Usefulness of Preoperative Laboratory Screening," *JAMA* 253(24):3576–3581, June 28, 1985.

Kennedy, R., Kennedy, M., et al., "Use of the Cardiac-Catheterization Laboratory in a Defined Population," *NEJM* 303(22):1273–1277, November 27, 1980.

Kent, D., and Larson, E., "Magnetic Resonance Imaging of the Brain and Spine: Is Clinical Efficacy Established After the First Decade?" *Annals of Internal Medicine* 108(3):402–424, 1988.

King, R., "Technology and the Doctor-Patient Relationship," *International Journal of Technology Assessment in Health Care* 3(1):11–18, 1987.

Knaus, W., and Wagner, D., "When Is ICU Care Appropriate?" *Business and Health*, pp. 31–34, January 1987.

Kosecoff, J., Chassin, M., et al., "Obtaining Clinical Data on the Appropriateness of Medical Care in Community Practice," *JAMA* 258(18):2538–2542, November 13, 1987.

Kralewski, J., Dowd, B., et al., "The Physician Rebellion," *NEJM* 316(6):339–342, February 5, 1987.

Kusserow, R., Handley, E., and Yessian, M., "An Overview of State Medical Discipline," *JAMA* 257(6):820–824, February 13, 1987.

Landfeld, S., Chren, M., et al., "Diagnostic Yield of the Autopsy in a University Hospital and a Community Hospital," *NEJM* 318(19):1249–1254, May 12, 1988.

Lasch, K., Maltz, A., et al., "A Protocol Approach to Assessing Medical Technologies," *International Journal of Technology Assessment in Health Care* 3(1):103–122, 1987.

Laudicina, S., "State Health Risk Pools: Insuring the 'Uninsurable'," *Health Affairs* 7(4):97–104, Fall 1988.

Leppert, P., and Namerow, "Costs Averted by Providing Comprehensive Prenatal Care to Teenagers," *Journal of Nurse-Midwifery* 30(5):285–289, September/October 1985.

Lohr, K., "Commentary: Professional Peer Review in a 'Competitive' Medical Market," *Case Western Reserve Law Review* 36(4):1175–1189, 1985–86.

Lomas, J., Anderson, G., et al., "The Role of Evidence in the Consensus Process," *JAMA* 259(20):3001–3005, May 27, 1988.

Luft, H., and Arno, P., "Impact of Increasing Physician Supply: A Scenario for the Future," *Health Affairs*, pp. 31–46, Winter 1986.

Luft, H., Bunker, J., and Enthoven, A., "Should Operations be Regionalized? The Empirical Relation between Surgical Volume and Mortality," *NEJM* 301:1364–1369, December 20, 1979.

Lynn, M., Waring, G., et al., "Factors Affecting Outcome and Predictability of Radial Keratotomy in the PERK Study," *Archives of Ophthalmology* 105:42–51, January 1987.

Massanari, R., Wilkerson, K., et al., "Reliability of Reporting Nosocomial Infections in the Discharge Abstract and Implications for Receipt of Revenues under Prospective Reimbursement," *American Journal of Public Health* 77(5):561–564, May 1987.

Masters, S., McClean, P., et al., "Skull X-Ray Examinations After Head Trauma," *NEJM* 316(2):84–91, January 8, 1987.

Mayer, W., Clinton, J., and Newhall, D., "A First Report of the Department of Defense External Civilian Peer Review of Medical Care," *JAMA* 260(18):2690–2693, November 11, 1988.

Mayes, F., Oakley, D., et al., "A Retrospective Comparison of Certified Nurse-Midwife and Physician Management of Low Births: A Pilot Study," *Journal of Nurse-Midwifery* 32(4):216–221, July/August 1987.

McCall, N., Rice, T., and Hall, A., "The Effect of State Regulations on the Quality and Sale of Insurance Policies to Medicare Beneficiaries," *Journal of Health Politics, Policy and Law* 12(1):53–76, Spring 1987.

McPherson, K., Wennberg, J., et al., "Small-Area Variations in the Use of Common Surgical Procedures: An International Comparison of New England, England, and Norway," *NEJM* 307(21):1310–1314, November 18, 1982.

Mechanic, D., "Challenges in Long-Term Care Policy," *Health Affairs* 6(2):22–33, Summer 1987.

"Medicaid Mill: Fact or Fiction," *Health Care Financing Review* 2(1):37–49, Summer 1980.

Meiners, M., "The Case for Long-Term Care Insurance," *Health Affairs* 2(2):56–79, Summer 1983.

Melnick, G., and Zwanziger, J., "Hospital Behavior Under Competition and Cost-Containment Policies: The California Experience, 1980 to 1985," *JAMA* 260(18):2669–2681, November 11, 1988.

Merrick, N., Brook, R., et al., "Use of Carotid Endarterectomy in Five California Veterans Administration Medical Centers," *JAMA* 256(18):2531–2535, November 14, 1986.

Myers, S., and Gleicher, N., "A Successful Program to Lower Cesarean-Section Rates," *NEJM* 319(23):1511–1516, December 8, 1988.

"News at Deadline," *Hospitals* 62(20):12, October 20, 1988 (reporting on a study reported in the October 3, 1988 edition of *Annals of Internal Medicine*).

Nycz, G., Wenzel, F., et al., "Medicare Risk Contracting: Lessons from an Unsuccessful Demonstration," *JAMA* 257(5):656–659, February 6, 1987.

Oberg, C., and Polich, C., "Medicaid: Entering the Third Decade," *Health Affairs* 7(4):83–95, Fall 1988.

O'Leary, D., "Quality Assessment: Moving from Theory to Practice," *JAMA* 260(12):1760, September 23/30, 1988.

Palmer, R., Strain, R., et al., "Quality Assurance in Eight Adult Medicine Group Practices," *Medical Care* 22(7):632–643, July 1984.

Panzer, R., and Griner, P., "Teaching Quantitative Approaches to the Use of Diagnostic Tests and Procedures," *International Journal of Technology Assessment in Health Care* 3(1):27–38, 1987.

Pasley, B., Vernon, P., et al., "Geographic Variations in Elderly Hospital and Surgical Discharge Rates, New York State," *American Journal of Public Health* 77(6):679–684, June 1987.

Pellegrino, E., "The Most Humane Science: Some Notes on Liberal Education in Medicine and the University," *Bulletin of the Medical College of Virginia* 67(4):11–39, Summer 1970.

Perlstadt, H., and Holmes, R., "The Role of Public Opinion Polling in Health Legislation," *American Journal of Public Health* 77(5):612–614, May 1987.

Perrin, J., and Valvona, J., "Does Increased Physician Supply Affect Quality of Care?" *Health Affairs*, pp. 63–72, Winter 1986.

Perry, S., and Wu, A., "Rationale for the Use of Hypnotic Agents in a General Hospital," *Annals of Internal Medicine* 100(3):441–446, March 1984.

Porkony, J., "Report on Health Care," *Health Management Quarterly* 10(1):5, 1988.

"Projection of Health Care Spending to 1990," *Health Care Financing Review* 7(3):1–35, Spring 1986, p. 2.

"PROs Use Medical Practice Standards to Assess Quality," *Hospitals* 62(20):19–20, October 20, 1988.

Reinhardt, U., "Quality: The Achilles' Heel of Market Strategy," *Hospitals*, p. 24, October 5, 1988.

Reinhardt, U., "Rationing Despite Surplus: A Paradox? or As American as Apple Pie?" *HealthSpan* 4(2):13–18, February 1987.

Reiss, J., Ward, D., and Bucci, V., "Rationing the Use of New Medical Technologies," *Topics in Health Law* 1(4):71–78, September 1986.

Relman, A., "Assessment and Accountability: The Third Revolution in Medical Care," *NEJM* 319(18):1220–1222, November 3, 1988.

Relman, A., "The Changing Climate of Medical Practice," *NEJM* 316(6):333–334, February 5, 1987.

Relman, A., "The Pressure to Keep Prices High at a Walk-in Clinic," *NEJM* 319(12):785–787, September 22, 1988.

Relman, A., "Salaried Physicians and Economic Incentives," *NEJM* 319(12):784, September 22, 1988.

Relman, A., and Reinhardt, U., "Debating For-Profit Health Care," *Health Affairs* 5(2):5–31, Summer 1986.

Restuccia, J., Gertman, P., et al., "A Comparative Analysis of Appropriateness of Hospital Use," *Health Affairs* 3(2):130–138, Summer 1984.

"Results of Second Opinion Program for Coronary Artery Bypass Graft Surgery," *Medical Benefits*, October 31, 1987.

Robinson, M., "Insurers, HMO Hit Big Recession in '87," *Hospitals*, pp. 27–28, September 5, 1988.

Robinson, M., "MD Malpractice Data Bank: Nobody's Happy," *Hospitals*, pp. 28–29, September 5, 1988.

Robinson, M., "Testing Guidelines Dropped as Reimbursement Tool," *Hospitals*, pp. 26–27, September 5, 1988.

Roe, B., "Rational Remuneration," *NEJM* 313(20):1286–1289, November 14, 1985.

Roe, B., "The UCR Boondoggle: A Death Knell for Private Practice?" *NEJM* 305(1):41–45, July 2, 1981.

Roos, L., Cageorge, S., and Danzinger, R., "Centralization, Certification, and Monitoring: Readmissions and Complications After Surgery," *Medical Care* 24(11):1044–1066, November 1986.

Roos, N., "Hysterectomy: Variations in Rates Across Small Areas and Across Physicians' Practices," *American Journal of Public Health* 74(4):327–335, April 1984.

Roper, W., "Perspectives on Physician-Patient Reform: The Resource-Based Relative-Value Scale in Context," *NEJM* 319(13):865–867, September 29, 1988.

Roper, W., Winkenwerder, W., et al., "Effectiveness in Health Care: An Initiative to Evaluate and Improve Medical Practice," *NEJM* 319(18):1197–1202, November 3, 1988.

Rosenfeld, K., Luft, H., and McPhee, S., "Changes in Patient Characteristics and Surgical Outcomes for Coronary Artery Bypass Surgery 1972–82," *American Journal of Public Health* 77(4):498–500, April 1987.

Rutkow, I., "Delivery of Surgical Health Care in the United States," *Archives of Surgery* 116:963–969, July 1981.

Rutkow, I., "General Surgical Operations in the United States, 1979 to 1984," *Archives of Surgery* 121:1145–1149, October 1986.

Rutkow, I., "Surgical Decision Making and Operative Rates," *Archives of Surgery* 119:899–905, August 1984.

Rutkow, I., "Surgical Operations in the United States: 1979 to 1984," *Surgery* 101(2):192–200, February 1987.

Rutkow, I., "Unnecessary Surgery: What Is It?" *Surgical Clinics of North America* 62(4):613–625, August 1982.

Sacks, H., Chalmers, T., and Reitman, D., "Should Mild Hypertension Be Treated? An Attempted Meta-Analysis of the Clinical Trials," *The Mount Sinai Journal of Medicine* 52(4):265–270, April 1985.

Sager, M., Leventhal, E., and Easterling, D., "The Impact of Medicare's Prospective Payment System on Wisconsin Nursing Homes," *JAMA* 257(13):1762–1766, April 3, 1987.

Sawitz, E., Showstack, J., et al., "The Use of In-Hospital Physician Services for Acute Myocardial Infarction: Changes in Volume and Complexity Over Time," *JAMA* 259(16):2419–2422, April 22/29, 1988.

Schroeder, S., "Strategies for Reducing Medical Costs by Changing Physicians' Behavior: Efficacy and Impact on Quality of Care," *International Journal of Technology Assessment in Health Care* 3(1):39–50, 1987.

Schroeder, S., and Martin, A., "Will Changing How Physicians Order Tests Reduce Medical Costs?" *Annals of Internal Medicine* 94(4.1):534–535, April 1981.

Schwartz, W., "The Inevitable Failure of Current Cost-Containment Strategies: Why They Can Provide Only Temporary Relief," *JAMA* 257(2):220–224, January 9, 1987.

Scovern, H., "Hired Help: A Physician's Experience in a For-Profit Staff-Model HMO," *NEJM* 319(12):787–790, September 22, 1988.

Scupholme, A., McLeod, A., and Robertson, E., "A Birth Center Affiliated with the Tertiary Care Center: Comparison of Outcome," *Obstetrics & Gynecology* 67(4):598–603, April 1986.

Selker, H., Griffith, J., et al., "How Do Physicians Adapt When the Coronary Care Unit Is Full?" *JAMA* 257(9):1181–1185, March 6, 1987.

Short, P., "Trends in Employee Health Benefits," *Health Affairs* 7(3):174–184, Summer 1988.

Showstack, J., Rosenfeld, K., et al., "Association of Volume with Outcome of Coronary Artery Bypass Graft Surgery," *JAMA* 257(6):785–789, February 13, 1987.

Siu, A., Sonnenberg, F., et al., "Inappropriate Use of Hospitals in a Randomized Trial of Health Insurance Plans," *NEJM* 315(20):1259–1266, November 13, 1986.

Slome, C., Wetherbee, H., et al., "Effectiveness of Certified Nurse-Midwives: A Prospective Evaluation Study," *American Journal of Obstetrics and Gynecology* 124(2):177–182, January 15, 1976.

Solovy, A., "RVS Will Bring Changes in Hospital Utilization," *Hospitals*, pp. 36, 40, September 5, 1988.

Starfield, B., "Motherhood and Apple Pie: The Effectiveness of Medical Care for Children," *Milbank Memorial Fund Quarterly/Health and Society* 63(3):523–546, 1985.

Steel, K., Gertman, P., et al., "Iatrogenic Illness on a General Medical Service at a University Hospital," *NEJM* 304(11):638–642, March 12, 1981.

Stokes III, J., "Why Not Rate Health and Life Insurance Premiums by Risks?" *NEJM* 308(7):393–395, February 17, 1983.

Thier, S., "Reexamining the Principles of Medicine," *Health Affairs* 6(4):70–74, Winter 1987.

Vayda, E., Mindell, W., and Rutkow, I., "A Decade of Surgery in Canada, England and Wales, and the United States," *Archives of Surgery* 117:846–852, June 1982.

Waring, G., "Making Sense of 'Keratospeak'," *Archives of Ophthalmology* 103:1472–1477, October 1985.

Waring, G., Lynn, M., et al., "Results of the Prospective Evaluation of Radial Keratotomy (PERK) Study One Year After Surgery," *Ophthalmology* 92(2):177–199, February 1985.

Weiner, J., Ehrenworth, D., and Spence, D., "Private Long-Term Care Insurance: Cost, Coverage, and Restrictions," *The Gerontologist* 27(4):487–493, 1987.

Wennberg, J., "Dealing with Medical Practice Variations: A Proposal for Action," *Health Affairs* 3(2):6–32, Summer 1984.

Wennberg, J., "Factors Governing Utilization of Hospital Services," *Hospital Practice* 14:115–121, 126–127, September 1979.

Wennberg, J., "Should the Cost of Insurance Reflect the Cost of Use in Local Hospital Markets?" *NEJM* 307(22):1374–1381, November 25, 1982.

Wennberg, J., and Gittelsohn, A., "Variations in Medical Care Among Small Areas," *Scientific American* 246:120–126, 129, 132, 134, April 1982.

Wennberg, J., Mulley, A., et al., "An Assessment of Prostatectomy for Benign Urinary Tract Obstruction: Geographic Variations and the Evaluation of Medical Care Outcomes," *JAMA* 259(20):3027–3030, May 27, 1988.

Wilensky, G., "Filling the Gaps in Health Insurance: Impact on Competition," *Health Affairs* 7(3):133–149, Summer 1988.

Winslow, C., Kosecoff, J., et al., "The Appropriateness of Performing Coronary Artery Bypass Surgery," *JAMA* 260(4):505–509, July 22/29, 1988.

Winslow, C., Solomon, D., et al., "The Appropriateness of Carotid Endarterectomy," *NEJM* 318(12):721–727, March 24, 1988.

Wong, E., and Lincoln, T., "Ready! Fire! . . . Aim!: An Inquiry into Laboratory Test Ordering," *JAMA* 250(18):2510–2513, November 11, 1983.

Yolles, B., Connors, J., and Grufferman, S., "Obtaining Access to Data from Government-Sponsored Medical Research," *NEJM* 315(26):1669–1672, December 25, 1986.

Zibrak, J., Rossetti, P., and Wood, E., "Effect of Reductions in Respiratory Therapy on Patient Outcome," *NEJM* 315(5):292–295, July 31, 1986.

Journal Editorials

Battaglia, F., "Reducing the Cesarean-Section Rate Safely," *NEJM* 319(23):1540–1541, December 8, 1988.

Blagg, C., "The End-Stage Renal Disease Program: Here Are Some of the Data," *JAMA* 257(5):662–663, February 6, 1987.

Breaden, D., and Galusha, B., "State Medical Discipline: Defects and Hindrances," *JAMA* 257(6):828–829, February 13, 1987.

Burnum, J., "Medical Vampires," *NEJM* 314(19):1250–1251, May 8, 1986.

Caper, P., "The Epidemiologic Surveillance of Medical Care," *American Journal of Public Health* 77(6):669–670, June 1987.

Caplan, L.R., "Carotid-Artery Disease," *NEJM* 315(14):886–889, October 2, 1986.

Chalmers, T., "PET Scans and Technology Assessment," *JAMA* 260(18):2713–2715, November 11, 1988.

DeWitt, T., "How Problematic Are Nosocomial Infections in the DRG Reimbursement System?" *American Journal of Public Health* 77(5):542–543, May 1987.

Feinstein, A., "On Classifying Cancers While Treating Patients," *Archives of Internal Medicine* 145(10):1789–1791, October 1985.

Fischer, H., "Cost vs. Safety: The Use of Low-Osmolar Contrast Media," *JAMA* 260(11):1614, September 16, 1988.

Jacoby, I., "Evidence and Consensus," *JAMA* 259(20):3039, May 27, 1988.

Johnson, K., "Beyond Tort Reform," *JAMA* 257(6):827–828, February 13, 1987.

Jonasson, O., and Barrett, J., "Transfer of Unstable Patients: Dumping or Duty?" *JAMA* 257(11):1519, March 20, 1987.

Kelly, J., "Assessing Quality," *JAMA* 260(18):2715–2716, November 11, 1988.

Lee, P., and Ginsburg, P., "Physician Payment Reform: An Idea Whose Time Has Come," *JAMA* 260(16):2441–2443, October 28, 1988.

Lundberg, G., "Acting on Significant Laboratory Results," *JAMA* 245(17):1763, May 1, 1981.

Lundberg, G., "Costs, Charges, Conscience, and Control (Lost)," *JAMA* 250(18):2509, November 11, 1983.

Lundberg, G., "Is There a Need for Routine Preoperative Laboratory Tests?" *JAMA* 253:3589, June 28, 1985.

Lundberg, G., "Medical Students, Truth, and Autopsies," *JAMA* 250(9):1199–1200, September 2, 1983.

Lundberg, G., "Perseveration of Laboratory Test Ordering: A Syndrome Affecting Clinicians," *JAMA* 249(5):639, February 4, 1983.

Lundberg, G., and Bodine, L., "Fifty Hours for the Poor," *JAMA* 260(21):3178, December 2, 1988.

Lundberg, G., and Westlake, G., "Cost Containment in the Clinical Laboratory—To Be or to Seem to Be, or When Is a Nontest a Test?" *JAMA* 243(16):1659, April 25, 1980.

McIntosh, H., "Second Opinions for Aortocoronary Bypass Grafting Are Beneficial," *JAMA* 258(12):1644–1645, September 25, 1987.

Mueller, C., "Surgery for Breast Cancer: Less May Be as Good as More," *NEJM* 312(11):712–714, March 14, 1985.

Mulley, Jr., A., and Eagle, K., "What Is Inappropriate Care?" *JAMA* 260(4):540–541, July 22/29, 1988.

O'Leary, D., "Quality Assessment: Moving from Theory to Practice," *JAMA* 260(12):1760, September 23/30, 1988.

Petty, T., "Rational Respiratory Therapy," *NEJM* 315(5):317–319, July 31, 1986.

Raisler, J., "Improving Pregnancy Outcome with Nurse-Midwifery Care," *Journal of Nurse-Midwifery* 30(4):189–192, July/August 1985.

Relman, A., "Assessment and Accountability: The Third Revolution in Medical Care," *NEJM* 319(18):1220–1222, November 3, 1988.

Roper, W., "The Resource-Based Relative-Value Scale: A Methodological and Policy Evaluation," *JAMA* 260(16):2444–2446, October 28, 1988.

Schroeder, S., "Outcome Assessment 70 Years Later: Are We Ready?" *NEJM* 316(3):160–162, January 15, 1987.

Spitzer, W., "The Nurse Practitioner Revisited: Slow Death of a Good Idea," *NEJM* 310(16):1049–1051, April 19, 1984.

Todd, J., "At Last, a Rational Way to Pay for Physicians' Services?" *JAMA* 260(16):2439–2441, October 28, 1988.

Vladeck, B., "Hospital Prospective Payment and the Quality of Care," *NEJM* 319(21):1411–1413, November 24, 1988.

Waring, G., "PERK Director Responds," *Journal of Refractive Surgery* 2(5):201–205, September/October 1986.

Waring, G., "Radial Keratotomy in Perspective," *American Journal of Ophthalmology* 92(2):286–291, August 1981.

Journal Correspondence

Boylan, P., "Electronic Fetal Monitoring and Cesarean Section," *NEJM* 316(8):480–481, February 19, 1987.

Carmichael, J., "The Cascade Effect in the Clinical Care of Patients," *NEJM* 315(5):319, July 31, 1986.

Chassin, M., Park, R., et al., "Variations in the Use of Medical and Surgical Services," *NEJM* 315(10):650, September 4, 1986.

Erlandson, J., and McCauley, C., "The Cascade Effect in the Clinical Care of Patients," *NEJM* 315(5):319, July 31, 1986.

Feldman, G., "Electronic Fetal Monitoring and Cesarean Section," *NEJM* 316(8):481–482, February 19, 1987.

Gardin, T., "Electronic Fetal Monitoring and Cesarean Section," *NEJM* 316(8):481, February 19, 1987.

Haynes de Regt, R., Minkoff, H., et al., "Electronic Fetal Monitoring and Cesarean Section," *NEJM* 316(8):482–483, February 19, 1987.

Kaufman, J., "Variations in the Use of Medical and Surgical Services," *NEJM* 315(10):649, September 4, 1986.

Kern, M., "The Cascade Effect in the Clinical Care of Patients," *NEJM* 315(5):319–320, July 31, 1986.

Leveno, K., and Cunningham, F., "Electronic Fetal Monitoring and Cesarean Section," *NEJM* 316(8):482, February 19, 1987.

Main, E., and Main, D., "Electronic Fetal Monitoring and Cesarean Section," *NEJM* 316(8):480, February 19, 1987.

Meier, P., "Electronic Fetal Monitoring and Cesarean Section," *NEJM* 316(8):481, February 19, 1987.

Mold, J., and Stein, H., "The Cascade Effect in the Clinical Care of Patients," *NEJM* 315(5):320, July 31, 1986.

Moore, F., "Variations in the Use of Medical and Surgical Services," *NEJM* 315(10):650–651, September 4, 1986.

Schor, E., and Grayson, M., "More on Diagnostic Restraint," *NEJM* 311(17):1128, October 25, 1984.

Scialli, A., "The Cascade Effect in the Clinical Care of Patients," *NEJM* 315(5):320, July 31, 1986.

Surgenor, D., and Hale, S., "Variations in the Use of Medical and Surgical Services," *NEJM* 315(10):649, September 4, 1986.

Weary, P., "Variations in the Use of Medical and Surgical Services," *NEJM* 315(10):649, September 4, 1986.

Wennberg, J., "Variations in the Use of Medical and Surgical Services," *NEJM* 315(10):650, September 4, 1986.

Newspaper Articles

Anderson, J., and Spear, J., "Eye Doctors See Millions in Medicare," *Washington Post*, September 10, 1985.

Bogdanich, W., "False Negative: Medical Labs, Trusted as Largely Error-Free, Are Far from Infallible," *Wall Street Journal*, February 2, 1987.

Bogdanich, W., "Labs Offering Workplace Drug Screens in New York Have Higher Error Rate," *Wall Street Journal*, February 2, 1987.

Bogdanich, W., "Risk Factor: Inaccuracy in Testing Cholesterol Hampers War on Heart Disease," *Wall Street Journal*, February 3, 1987.

Cohen, T., "The High Cost of Bad Medicine," *Washington Post*, September 20, 1983.

Cohn, V., "Hospitalization Found Dangerous to Your Health," *Washington Post*, March 15, 1981.

Eckholm, E., "Problems After Myopia Surgery Cited in Study," *New York Times*, October 1, 1985.

Engel, M., "Evaluation of Ovarian Cancer Faulted," *Washington Post*, June 20, 1985.

Engel, M., "$2 Billion Lost to Eye Doctors, Hill Panel Says," *Washington Post*, July 16, 1985.

Hilts, P., "New Study Faults Hospital Monitoring of Fetal Heartbeats," *Washington Post*, January 11, 1981.

Rich, S., "Medicare Fees May Reward Extra Surgery," *Washington Post*, December 7, 1985.

Robin, E., "Surgery for Nearsighted Eyes Is a High-Stakes Gamble," *Washington Post*, October 30, 1985.

Russell, C., "Breast Cancer Death Rate Up for Younger Women," *Washington Post*, December 8, 1986.

Russell, C., "Study Casts Doubt on Cancer Statistics," *Washington Post*, June 20, 1985.

Russell, C., "Study Suggests Overuse of Intensive Care Units," *Washington Post*, December 16, 1981.

Sinclair, M., "Prices 32% Lower Where Optometrists Advertise," *Washington Post*, May 16, 1980.

"Study Cites Misdiagnoses," *Washington Post*, April 28, 1984.

BOOKS AND CHAPTERS

Bovbjerg, R., *Facilitating Health Care Coverage for the Working Uninsured: Alternative State Strategies*, Health Policy Studies, Center for Policy Research, National Governors' Association, Washington, DC, September 1987.

Donabedian, A., *The Methods and Findings of Quality Assessment and Monitoring: An Illustrated Analysis, Vol. III*, Health Administration Press, Ann Arbor, Michigan, 1985.

Eisenberg, J., *Doctors' Decisions and the Cost of Medical Care*, Health Administration Press, Ann Arbor, MI, 1986.

Etheredge, L., Reinhardt, U., et al., "Hard Choices in Health Care: A Matter of Ethics," *Health Care: How to Improve It and Pay for It*, Center for National Policy, Washington, DC, April 1985.

Feinstein, A., *Clinical Judgement*, Williams and Wilkins Company, Baltimore, 1967. Reprinted, Robert E. Creiger Publishing Company, Huntington, NY, 1974.

Ginsburg, P., and Sunshine, J., *Cost Management in Employee Health Plans*, RAND, Supported by the Robert Wood Johnson Foundation, R-3543-RWJ, October 1987.

Institute of Medicine, *Assessing Medical Technologies*, National Academy Press, Washington, DC, 1985.

Institute of Medicine, *The Future of Public Health*, National Academy Press, Washington, DC, 1988.

Institute of Medicine, *Improving the Quality of Care in Nursing Homes*, National Academy Press, Washington, DC, 1986.

Institute of Medicine, *Medical Technology Assessment Directory*, National Academy Press, Washington, DC, 1988.

Institute of Medicine, *Preventing Low Birthweight*, National Academy Press, Washington, DC, 1985.

Institute of Medicine, *Quality of Care and Technology Assessment: Report of a Forum of* the Council on Health Care Technology, National Academy Press: Washington, DC, 1988.

Isaacs, J., editor, For-Profit & Nonprofit Health Care: Are the Distinctions Blurring? National Health Council, Inc., March 1987.

Litan, R., and Winston, C., editors, Liability Perspectives and Policy, The Brookings Institution, Washington, DC, 1988.

Manning, W., Newhouse, J., et al., Health Insurance and the Demand for Medical Care: Evidence from a Randomized Experiment, RAND Research Report, R 3476 HHS, February 1988.

Rosou, J., and Zayer, R., Improving Health Care Management in the Workplace, Pergamon Press: Elmsford, NY, 1985.

Rother, J., Gibson, M., and Varner, T., Catastrophic and Long-Term Care Costs: A Closer Look, American Association of Retired Persons, Washington, DC, 1987.

Rubin, R., Moran, D., et al., Critical Condition: America's Health Care in Jeopardy, National Committee for Quality Health Care, Washington, DC, 1988.

Solomon, D., Brook, R., et al., Indications for Selected Medical and Surgical Procedures—A Literature Review and Ratings of Appropriateness: Cholecystectomy, The RAND Publication Series, R-3204/3-CWF/HF/PMT/RWJ, ISBN 0-8330-0743-2, May 1986.

SPECIAL REPORT, Access to Health Care in the United States: Results of a 1986 Survey, The Robert Wood Johnson Foundation, Number 2, 1987.

Thompson, J.E., "Nurse Midwifery Care: 1925 to 1984," Annual Review of Nursing Research, pp. 153–173, Werley, H., Fitzpatrick, J., and Taunton, R. (eds.), Springer Publishing Company, New York, 1986.

University of Chicago, Graduate Program in Health Administration and Center for Health Administration Studies, Graduate School of Business, Division of Biological Sciences, Cost Containment and Physician Autonomy: Implications for Quality of Care, Proceedings of the Twenty-Eighth Annual George Bugbee Symposium on Hospital Affairs, May 1986.

Wilensky, G., "Solving Uncompensated Hospital Care," in M.B. Sulvetta and K. Swartz (eds), The Uninsured and Uncompensated Care: A Chartbook, National Health Policy Forum, George Washington University, Washington, DC, June 1986.

UNPUBLISHED MATERIALS

Altman, S., "The American Healthcare System: The Twilight Zone Between Competition and Regulation," Emerging Issues in Health Care, Estes Park Institute, Englewood, CA, 1988.

American Medical Association, Professional Liability Clearinghouse Holdings, an annotated bibliography, May/July/August through October/December 1986, March 1987.

Beach Hall, statement to National Leadership Commission on Health Care, March 18, 1988.

Berwick, D., "Measuring Health Care Quality," unpublished paper MS# PR40-87/88, Harvard Community Health Plan, September 21, 1987.

Blue Cross and Blue Shield Association, "Anti-Fraud Press Conference," Washington, DC, December 10, 1986.

Butler, R., "Life After Cost Containment: Perspectives on Meeting the Health Care Needs of Older People," prepared for the Anglo-American Conference on *Need, Demand and Resources: Health Care Provision at a Time of Financial Restraint*, The Royal Society of Medicine, London, December 2–4, 1986.

Chalmers, T., and Berk, A., "The Relative Costs of Diseases, Ineffective and Effective Therapies, and Randomized Control Trials (1)," testimony before the Subcommittee on Health and Long Term Care of the U.S. House of Representatives Select Committee on Aging, March 15, 1984.

Chassin, M., *Standards of Care in Medicine*, prepared for the Health Industry Manufacturers' Association Health Policy Seminar, Woods Hole, MA, August 1988.

Chollet, D., "Quality of Care as a Constraint on Cost Containment in the Private Sector," draft, for presentation at the annual meeting of the American Public Health Association, New Orleans, LA, October 20, 1987.

Danzon, P., "The Effects of Tort Reforms on the Frequency and Severity of Medical Malpractice Claims: A Summary of Research Results," The Institute for Civil Justice, The RAND Corporation, testimony submitted to the Committee on the Judiciary, U.S. Senate, March 26, 1986.

Donabedian, A., "The Price of Quality and the Perplexities of Care," the 1986 Michael M. Davis Lecture, The Center for Health Administration Studies, Graduate School of Business, Division of Biological Sciences, University of Chicago, May 9, 1986.

Dukakis, M., *Statement on New Massachusetts Health Partnership: Health Care for All*, August 13, 1987.

Eddy, D., and Billings, J., "The Quality of Medical Evidence and Practice," a paper produced for the National Leadership Commission on Health Care, May 1987.

Enthoven, A., *A Consumer Choice Health Plan for the 1990s: A Proposal for Universal Health Insurance*, February 3, 1988.

Fink, A., Brook, R., et al., "The Sufficiency of the Clinical Literature for Learning About the Appropriate Uses of Six Medical and Surgical Procedures," The Departments of Economics and System Sciences at The RAND Corporation, Center for the Health Sciences, Santa Monica, California and Departments of Medicine and Public Health at the University of California, Los Angeles, unpublished draft, 1987.

Frech, H., and Ginsburg, P., "Competition Among Health Insurers: Revisited," January 5, 1988, originally published in *Competition in the Health Sector: Past, Present, and Future* (Washington, DC, Federal Trade Commission, 1978).

Griner, P., "AMA Inaugural Medical Staff Conference (Quality Assurance)," presentation, October 1985.

Louis Harris and Associates, *Making Difficult Health Care Decisions*, Massachusetts, The Loran Commission, June 1987. Cited in Daniel Callahan, "Allocating Health Resources," *Hastings Center Report*, April/May, 1988.

Keller, R., statement before the U.S. Senate Committee on Finance, Subcommittee on Health, July 11, 1988.

Lewin/ICF, Inc., *Expenditures and Revenues Under an Illustrative Universal Health Coverage Plan*, prepared for the National Leadership Commission on Health Care, September 27, 1988.

Lewin, L., "Cost Containment Until Today: Lessons for Tomorrow," paper prepared for the National Leadership Commission on Health Care, May 1988.

Lipson, D., and Fisher, R., *Major Changes in State Medicaid and Indigent Care Programs, January–December 1986*, compiled by the Intergovernmental Health Policy Project, The George Washington University.

Meiners, M., "Long-Term Care Insurance," *HCAM Convention*, September 1987.

Meyer, J., testimony before the National Economic Commission, October 19, 1988.

Moskowitz, G., Mak, N., et al., "Good Technology and Poor Clinical Science: Evaluation of Abdominal Imaging Procedures," portions of this work were presented at the meeting of the Association of American Physicians, Washington, DC, May 1983.

National Bureau of Standards, "Applications Guidelines 1988: Malcolm Baldridge National Quality Award."

Phillips, R., HCFA, letter to Simmons, H., National Leadership Commission on Health Care, October 13, 1988.

President's Commission for the Study of Ethical Problems in Medicine and Biomedical and Behavioral Research, *Securing Access to Health Care: A Report on the Ethical Implication of Differences in the Availability of Health Services,* March 1983.

Public Policy Options to Expand Health Insurance Coverage Among the Nonelderly Population, EBRI Issue Brief, Number 67, June 1987.

Reinhardt, U., "Decision-Making, Control and Implementation of Resource Allocation: The Resource Transfer from Patients to Providers of Health Services," paper prepared for the Anglo-American Conference, The Royal Society of Medicine, London, December 2–4, 1986.

Robinson, J., Luft, H., et al., "Hospital Competition and Surgical Length of Stay," unpublished research supported by grant number HS 05376-01 from the National Center for Health Services Research, U.S. Department of Health and Human Services, March 1987.

Roos, L., and Cageorge, S., "Choices, Efficiency and Outcomes: Research Strategies Using Claims," Faculties of Management and Medicine, University of Manitoba, unpublished paper, 1986.

S. 1265. *Minimum Health Benefits for All Workers Act* (Senators Edward M. Kennedy and Lowell P. Weiker).

S. 1370 and S. 1386. *Summary. Health Insurance Protection for the Self-Employed* (Senators Dale Bumpers and Edward M. Kennedy).

Shapiro, M., personal communication to Campbell, P., The Lash Group.

Swain, F., statement before the Committee on Labor and Human Resources of the U.S. Senate, "Mandated Employer-Paid Health Insurance, S. 1265," June 24, 1987.

U.S. Congress, Office of Technology Assessment, "Research on Geographic Variations in Physician Practice Patterns," Staff Paper, February 1987.

U.S. Congressional Budget Office, "Profile of Health Care Coverage: The Haves and Have-Nots," background paper, March 1979.

Webber, A., testimony before the U.S. Senate Committee on Finance, Subcommittee on Health, July 11, 1988.

Weiner, J., *We Can Run, But We Can't Hide: Financing Options for Long-Term Care,* Testimony before Budget Committee, U.S. House of Representatives, on "Long-Term Care of the Elderly," October 1, 1987.

Weiner, J., Hanley, R., et al., *Financing and Organizational Options for Long-Term Care,* testimony before Subcommittee on Health, Ways and Means Committee, U.S. House of Representatives, on "Long-Term Care," March 31, 1987.

Wennberg, J., "The Medical Care Outcome Problem: An Agenda for Action," paper prepared for the National Leadership Commission on Health Care, May 1987.

Wennberg, J., testimony before the U.S. Senate Committee on Finance, Subcommittee on Health, July 11, 1988.

GOVERNMENT PUBLICATIONS

Federal Register, Health Care Financing Administration, "Medicare Program: Changes to the Inpatient Prospective Payment System and Fiscal Year 1986 Rates; Proposed Rules," June 10, 1985, pp. 24366–24497.

Prospective Payment Assessment Commission, *Medicare Prospective Payment and the American Health Care System: Report to the Congress,* U.S. Government Printing Office, Washington, DC, June 1988.

U.S. Congress, Congressional Research Service, Library of Congress, *CRS Report for Congress—Catastrophic Health Insurance: Comparison of the Major Provision of the "Medicare Catastrophic Act of 1987"* (H.R. 2470 *as passed by the House, July 22, 1987) and the "Medicare Catastrophic Loss Prevention Act of 1987"* (H.R. 2470 *as passed by the Senate, October 27, 1987),* by Jennifer O'Sullivan and Janet Lundy, Education and Public Welfare Division 87-948 EPW, Library of Congress, Washington, DC, Revised February 24, 1988.

U.S. Congress, Congressional Research Service, Library of Congress, *Major Issues System Issue Brief—Catastrophic Health Insurance: Medicare,* by Jennifer O'Sullivan, Education and Public Welfare Division IB87106, Library of Congress, Washington, DC, Updated, February 25, 1988.

U.S. Congress, Congressional Research Service, Library of Congress, *Major Issues System Issue Brief—Medicare: Physician Payments,* by Jennifer O'Sullivan, Education and Public Welfare Division IB85007, Library of Congress, Washington, DC, Updated, February 8, 1988.

U.S. Congress, Office of Technology Assessment, *Medical Technology and Costs of the Medicare Program,* OTA-H-227, U.S. Government Printing Office, Washington, DC, July 1984.

U.S. Congress, Office of Technology Assessment, *Medicare's Prospective Payment System: Strategies for Evaluating Cost, Quality, and Medical Technology,* OTA-H-262, U.S. Government Printing Office, Washington, DC, October 1985.

U.S. Congress, Office of Technology Assessment, *Payment for Physician Services: Strategies for Medicare,* OTA-H-294, U.S. Government Printing Office, Washington, DC, February 1986.

U.S. Department of Health and Human Services, Health Care Financing Administration, *Health Care Financing: Program Statistics, Medicare and Medicaid Databook, 1986,* Publication 03247, September 1987, pp. 21–29.

U.S. Department of Health and Human Services, National Center for Health Statistics, *Detailed Diagnosis and Procedures for Patients Discharged from Short-stay Hospitals, United States, 1985,* Series 13(90), Publication 87-1751, April 1987.

U.S. Department of Health and Human Services, Office of Inspector General, *Medical Licensure and Discipline: An Overview,* Control Number P-01-86-00064, Region I, Boston, MA, June 1986.

U.S. Department of Health and Human Services, Office of Inspector General, *Semiannual Report to the Congress: April 1, 1986–September 30, 1986.*

U.S. Department of Health and Human Services, Office of Inspector General, *OIG Strategic Work Plan Fiscal Years 1987/1988,* draft mimeo, 1987.

U.S. Department of Health and Human Services, Public Health Service, Office of the Assistant Secretary for Health, Wennberg, J., Principal Investigator, *Small Area Variations in Hospitalized Case Mix for DRGs in Maine, Massachusetts and Iowa,* NCHSR Grant HS-04932, October 31, 1984.

U.S. Department of Health and Human Services, *Report to Congress and the Secretary,* Task Force on Long-Term Health Care Policies, September 21, 1987.

U.S. Department of Labor, Bureau of Labor Statistics, *Employee Benefits in Medium and Large Firms, 1985*, U.S. Government Printing Office, 029-001-02903-9, 1986.

U.S. General Accounting Office, Report to the Chairman, Subcommittee on Health and Long-Term Care, Select Committee on Aging, House of Representatives, *Long-Term Care Insurance: Coverage Varies Widely in a Developing Market*, GAO/HRD 87-80, May 1987.

U.S. General Accounting Office, Report to the Ranking Minority Member, Committee on Veterans' Affairs, U.S. Senate, *VA Health Care—VA's Patient Injury Control Program Not Effective*, GAO/HRD-87-49, May 1987.

U.S. General Accounting Office, Report to the Ranking Minority Member, Special Committee on Aging, U.S. Senate, *Medicare: Improved Patient Outcome Analyses Could Enhance Quality Assessment*, GAO/PEMD-88-23, June 1988.

U.S. General Accounting Office, Report to the Ranking Minority Member, Special Committee on Aging, U.S. Senate, *VA Hospital Care: A Comparison of VA and HCFA Methods for Analyzing Patient Outcomes*, GAO/PEMD-88-29, June 1988.

U.S. House of Representatives, 100th Congress, Second Session, A Report of the Select Committee on Children, Youth, and Families, *Opportunities for Success: Cost Effective Programs for Children, Update, 1988*, U.S. Government Printing Office, Washington, DC, 1988.